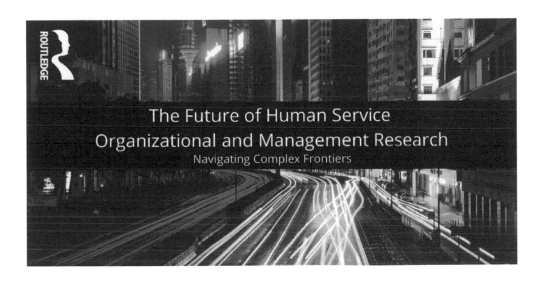

The Future of Human Service
Organizational and Management Research
Navigating Complex Frontiers

ROUTLEDGE

The Future of Human Service Organizational & Management Research

This book provides panoramic overviews of critical human service organizational and management practice challenges, as well as new and needed research frontiers.

The Future of Human Service Organizational & Management Research: Navigating Complex Frontiers invites researchers, educators, and practitioners to explore: the intersection of the complex environment of public and private human service organizations, and the rise and uncertain effects of new developments in social work, public policy and public management, and other helping professions. The contributors identify how future generations of macro practitioners and scholar-researchers can:

- Improve service delivery and program effectiveness;
- Implement evidence-based practices and evidence-informed practices;
- Promote leadership and social innovation;
- Build linkages across micro, meso, and macro levels of practice;
- Train organizational leaders and educate practitioners; and
- Advocate for more socially just visions of social welfare and society.

This edited collection argues that human service organizational and management practice and research are needed to support new discoveries in social welfare, social work, and related professions.

This book was originally published as a special issue of the journal *Human Service Organizations: Management, Leadership & Governance.*

Bowen McBeath is a Professor in the School of Social Work and Hatfield School of Government at Portland State University, USA.

Karen Hopkins is an Associate Professor in the School of Social Work at the University of Maryland, College Park, USA.

The Future of Human Service Organizational & Management Research

Navigating Complex Frontiers

Edited by
Bowen McBeath and Karen Hopkins

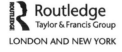

Routledge
Taylor & Francis Group

LONDON AND NEW YORK

First published 2020
by Routledge
2 Park Square, Milton Park, Abingdon, Oxon, OX14 4RN

and by Routledge
52 Vanderbilt Avenue, New York, NY 10017

Routledge is an imprint of the Taylor & Francis Group, an informa business

British Library Cataloguing-in-Publication Data
A catalogue record for this book is available from the British Library

ISBN13: 978-0-367-48481-1
ISBN13: 978-0-367-49532-9 (pbk)

Typeset in Minion Pro
by codeMantra

Publisher's Note
The publisher accepts responsibility for any inconsistencies that may have arisen during the conversion of this book from journal articles to book chapters, namely the inclusion of journal terminology.

Disclaimer
Every effort has been made to contact copyright holders for their permission to reprint material in this book. The publishers would be grateful to hear from any copyright holder who is not here acknowledged and will undertake to rectify any errors or omissions in future editions of this book.

Contents

Citation Information

The chapters in this book were originally published in *Human Service Organizations: Management, Leadership & Governance*, volume 43, issue 4 (September–October 2019). When citing this material, please use the original page numbering for each article, as follows:

Human Service Organizations: Management, Leadership & Governance, volume 43, issue 4 (September–October 2019) pp. 344–356

Chapter 11
Crafting the Future of Macro Practice
John Tropman and Bowen McBeath
Human Service Organizations: Management, Leadership & Governance, volume 43, issue 4 (September–October 2019) pp. 357–365

For any permission-related enquiries please visit:
http://www.tandfonline.com/page/help/permissions

Contributors

Michael J. Austin, School of Social Welfare, University of California, Berkeley, USA.

Michàlle E. Mor Barak, Suzanne Dworak-Peck School of Social Work, University of Southern California, Los Angeles, USA.

Alicia C. Bunger, College of Social Work, The Ohio State University, Columbus, USA.

Lauri Goldkind, Graduate School of Social Service, Fordham University, New York City, USA.

Richard Hoefer, School of Social Work, University of Texas at Arlington, Arlington, USA.

Karen Hopkins, School of Social Work, University of Maryland, Baltimore, USA.

Rebecca Lengnick-Hall, Brown School, Washington University in St. Louis, USA.

Nicole P. Marwell, School of Social Service Administration, University of Chicago, USA.

Bowen McBeath, School of Social Work and Hatfield School of Government (Division of Public Administration), Portland State University, USA.

Jenifer Huang McBeath, College of Natural Sciences and Mathematics, University of Alaska, Fairbanks, USA.

John G. McNutt, Biden School of Public Policy and Administration, University of Delaware, Newark, USA.

Megan Meyer, School of Social Work, University of Maryland, Baltimore, USA.

Jennifer E. Mosley, School of Social Service Administration, University of Chicago, USA.

Sunggeun (Ethan) Park, School of Social Work, University of Michigan, Ann Arbor, USA.

Rogério M. Pinto, School of Social Work, University of Michigan, Ann Arbor, USA.

Anna Maria Santiago, School of Social Work, Michigan State University, East Lansing, USA.

Richard J. Smith, School of Social Work, Wayne State University, Detroit, USA.

Qing Tian, Environmental Education Center, Faculty of Education, Beijing Normal University, P. R. of China.

John Tropman, School of Social Work and Ross School of Business, University of Michigan, Ann Arbor, USA.

Bin Xu, MSW Center, School of Humanities and Social Sciences, University of Science and Technology-Beijing, P. R. of China.

Marci Ybarra, School of Social Service Administration, University of Chicago, USA.

Gratitude and Dedication

Bowen McBeath and Karen Hopkins

The special issue began with a series of conversations that coincided with our assumption of the co-editorship of the journal. In our discussions, we were excited to find a special issue *topic* and an *approach* to the special issue that would reflect our interest in connecting the present world of human service organizational and management practice with the future-forward world of research on human service organizations and managers.

The topic of "The Future of Human Service Organizational and Management Research" was thus quite easy to select. We were interested in having leading scholars provide panoramic overviews of critical human service organizational and management practice challenges and needed future research emphases. We were not at all interested in restricting the topic to a well-defined subfield of human service organizations and management; nor did we want to be dogmatic in how authors approached their pieces. In essence, our hope was that the authors of the 10 commentaries comprising the special issue would offer their own perspectives, using their own scholarly styles and research backgrounds, to contribute to the good of the whole.

The approach was a little more challenging to envision, but soon took flight as we played with the idea of a macro practice/research salon. To Habermas as well as critical scholars of the Enlightenment era, salons emerged in Europe as rising economic conditions supported the development of bourgeois social cultures. (A comparable institution in Asia was organized around teahouses.) Salons were small, intimate gatherings that sought to promote high-level dialogue and sharing of the newest ideas, while drawing connections to classical influences. They presented opportunities for serious and convivial discussion, in which guests were intimately connected with current affairs because they were deeply involved in them. Needless to say, there was a performative aspect to the salon, involving intellectual interchanges that were rooted in the concerns of the present.

Salons arguably fell into disuse as a result of reduced cosmopolitanism and increased nationalism and authoritarianism. The idea of a macro practice/research salon therefore appealed to us, as it reflected: the need to identify and support future generations of macro practitioners and scholar-researchers; the rise and uncertain effects of new research and educational developments in the social work academy; and the changing environment of public and private human service organizations. The macro practice/research salon thus provided an opportunity for the commentators to make individual and collective sense of these developments.

We express our immense gratitude to those who supported the salon. In their capacity as current and former Managing Editor of the journal, Amanda Mosby and Tiffany Newton were indispensable in organizing the salon and seeing the special issue through to its completion. Abby Carson from Taylor & Francis supported the food and beverages so needed for our gathering. And Patty Couch of Travelink and the Society for Social Work and Research provided the venue for the salon.

After the salon concluded, the following experts helped to improve the works-in-progress as the special issue took shape. We name them here to express our gratitude for their efforts.

Mike Austin, University of California-Berkeley.
Kristina Jaskyte Bahr, University of Georgia.
Stephanie Berzin, Simmons University.
Alicia Bunger, The Ohio State University.
Philip Gillingham, University of Queensland.
Lauri Goldkind, Fordham University.
Geetha Gopalan, The City University of New York.
Erick Guerrero, University of Southern California.

Anna Haley, Rutgers, The State University of New Jersey.
Susan Lambert, University of Chicago.
Jennifer Mosley, University of Chicago.
Tom Packard, San Diego State University.
Hillel Schmid, The Hebrew University of Jerusalem.
Micheal Shier, University of Toronto.
Brenda Smith, University of Alabama.
Michael Spencer, University of Washington.
Rebecca Wells, University of Texas.
Allison Zippay, Rutgers, The State University of New Jersey.

We conclude with a note of deep appreciation to Mike Austin. Mike was a consistent and gracious presence by our side as our early conversations evolved into the macro practice/research salon and the special issue. Mike also contributed directly to the special issue with his own commentary. His indirect and direct contributions reflect his enthusiasm for human service organizational and management research, his investments in the journal and in macro social work, and his commitment to current and future generations of educators and scholars. We dedicate this special issue to him.

Navigating Complex Frontiers: Introduction to the Special Issue on "The Future of Human Service Organizational and Management Research"

Bowen McBeath and Karen Hopkins

ABSTRACT
Research on human service organizations and managers is essential and is needed to support both practice and scholarship. In response to a proposed imbalance between the two (between what we do and what we know), this special issue presents 10 commentaries that identify longstanding practice dilemmas and suggest new avenues for practice and research in social work and related helping professions and disciplines. Review of the commentaries supports three interrelated themes: (1) increasing complexity facing the environment of practice; leading to (2) proposed approaches to managing complexity across levels of practice; resulting in (3) implications for the future of macro practice, research, and education. The introduction concludes with a brief reflection on the future of human service organizational and management research. The overall aim of our analysis and the special issue is to illuminate that which is often hidden in plain view.

This special issue on "The Future of Human Service Organizational and Management Research" invites researchers, educators, and practitioners to explore questions at the intersection of human service organizations and management (HSO&M). These questions concern how to: improve service delivery and program effectiveness; promote leadership and social innovation at different levels of practice; train leaders and educate practitioners; and advocate for more socially just visions of social welfare and society. Historically, questions concerning HSO&M have coincided with the rise of the social work profession, as organizational and management scholarship has been used to understand and improve the lives of poor, at-risk peoples and communities. These questions are therefore of historic importance to practitioners and researchers in social work, the helping professions, and the social science disciplines.

The 10 commentaries comprising the special issue support varied understandings of human services. However, the commentaries reflect two shared premises. First, they posit that HSO&M practice and research are essential, and are increasingly needed to support new discoveries in social welfare, social work, and related professions. Second, the commentaries provide affirmative arguments concerning the future of macro practice research and scholarship in social work and related professions. Operationally, the aim of the special issue is to unearth and illuminate that which is essential-yet-hidden, often in plain view.

Each of the commentaries contributes to this aim, as follows:

(1) Michael Austin identifies three pathways for promoting macro practice in social work education.
(2) Alicia Bunger and Rebecca Lengnick-Hall propose collaborative research strategies involving implementation science and human service organizational researchers.
(3) Lauri Goldkind and John McNutt identify essential skills and training needs of human service leaders as they transition from managing programs to managing information ecosystems.

(4) Richard Hoefer proposes four Modest Challenges that are needed to ensure that social workers can address Grand Challenges.
(5) Karen Hopkins and Megan Meyer provide a novel framework and practical strategies for evaluating behavioral and organizational outcomes of leadership development in human service organizations.
(6) Bowen McBeath, Qing Tian, Bin Xu, and Jenifer Huang McBeath offer a vision of macro practice, education, research, and theory that is rooted in environmental justice and HSO&M.
(7) Michalle Mor Barak presents a theory-informed framework that is located in the concept of social good and that expands the horizons of macro social work and HSO&M research across sectors for positive social impact.
(8) Jennifer Mosley, Nicole Marwell, and Marci Ybarra identify challenges to the What Works movement and offer alternatives centered in organizational learning, consumer involvement, and community-based knowledge development.
(9) Rogerio Pinto and Sunggeun Park distinguish between the implementation and de-implementation of evidence-based practices (EBPs) and offer research evidence and theory in support of a framework of EBP de-implementation.
(10) Anna Maria Santiago and Richard Smith chart promising directions for human service professionals and community leaders who seek to use Big Data to address accountability concerns.

The special issue thus arrives at a propitious time, as scholars are taking HSO&M more seriously. Our introduction to the special issue is organized as follows. The next section provides a basic context for research on HSO&M. We then describe the process used to invite commentaries, and we introduce the 10 commentaries properly. We follow with an integrative review of themes from the commentaries. We conclude with a brief reflection on the future of human service organizational and management research.

The context for the special issue

To set the stage, we begin by defining HSO&M. For the purposes of the special issue, human service organizations reflect the following attributes: (a) they mostly focus upon assisting people, particularly those who are poor; (b) they depend upon institutionalized market environment for needed resources and legitimacy, and thus engage in interorganizational collaboration and competition; (c) their responses to external challenges often result in working conditions characterized by complexity, ambiguity, and discretion; (d) their organizing of service programs and structuring of assistance is highly indeterminate and involves moral work; and (e) at the frontline level, service delivery involves worker-service user relationships that are political, gendered, and involve emotional labor (Hasenfeld, 2010). The management of human services can refer to those "informed and competent responses to internal and external demands" (Menefee, 2009, p. 101) that are needed to improve service delivery, collaboration, and performance (Patti, 2009).

Historically, human service organizations have included commonly understood organizations such as public and private (mostly nonprofit) social welfare agencies as well as hospitals and schools (Hasenfeld, 1983). Management of these formal organizations has generally involved the following three practice domains (with managerial roles in parentheses): analytical (leveraging resources, managing resources, policy practice, evaluation); interactional (communicating, facilitating, supervising, advocating); and leadership (teaming, aligning, boundary spanning, and envisioning/futuring) (Austin, 2018; Menefee, 2009). The basic expectation connecting HSO&M to practice and programming is that effective management is needed to operate human service organizations effectively.

Our special issue focuses squarely on public and private social welfare agencies. However, all commentators are situated within schools of social work, and many of the commentaries specifically concern social work education and training in relation to the complex interorganizational ecology of human service organizations. Schools of social work are arguably a special type of human service organization, and deans and directors are essential for their management and leadership (Adedoyin, Miller, Jackson, Dodor, & Hall, 2016; Call, Owens, & Vincent, 2013). In the second-to-last section of our introductory paper, we therefore highlight the importance of deans and directors providing sufficient resources to connect micro, meso, and macro levels of practice.

The purposes of research on human service organizations and management

As conceived by this journal, HSO&M research has traditionally used social science methods to address organizational and management questions to respond to societal dilemmas effectively and ethically. The inaugural editor of the journal, Si Slavin, noted:

> "It is our intention to further the development and understanding of the processes, principles, and practices of administration and management in the social and human services. The journal will focus interest on theory, research, and practice, with special attention to the relationship between social administration and social policy planning. Its constituency will consist of executives, sub-executives, and middle managers in service-providing organizations. Its concern will be with values as well as technology, with normative and empirical studies, with the integrity of client service delivery as well as accountability and evaluation. To these ends, we invite manuscripts from persons in related professions in the network of social service systems" (1977, p. 3).

Basic foci of the journal have remained stable over its 43 years of operation. Our research emphases have also been consistent in studying the management, leadership, and governance dimensions of human service organizations including:

- Implications associated with the strings attached to traditional and new funding sources, policies and their implementation, and community-based dynamics.
- Issues of organizational performance, effectiveness, equity, and quality.
- Strategic planning, interorganizational and intra-organizational collaboration, and organizational change tactics.
- The involvement of managers and leaders in stewarding organizations and supporting programs and enterprises.
- The structuring and improvement of team-based work at all levels of the organization.
- Workforce development through competency-based education and training.
- Efforts to advocate internally and externally while trying to reconcile business management practices with the principles of human dignity.
- Initiatives to reduce the research-to-practice gap and enhance knowledge development and translation.

In regards to the application of research to support practice, the epistemological and methodological approaches used have been eclectic and diverse, although they have generally affirmed questions centered in organizational and managerial life. HSO&M research can therefore be viewed as a practical strategy for building, supporting, sharing, mobilizing, advocating, and defending. For example, in Issue 2 of the inaugural volume of this journal, Harold Lewis (then Dean and Professor at Hunter College School of Social Work – City University of New York) argued that the future role of human service managers in an "age of accountability" (1977, p. 116) would involve responding to continuing charges of poor performance by demonstrating knowledge of management competencies and service technologies, and by using management-by-objective and other business practices to legitimize program efforts in the face of substantial ambiguity. Lewis's reflections upon the Nixon and Ford administrations were prescient; and research on HSO&M has remained a critical strategy for shielding human service organizations and service users. The idea that HSO&M research should contribute directly and/or indirectly to practice is thus a bedrock principle of our journal.

HSO&M research is also critical for applied scholarship and theory. First, research helps scholars understand how HSO&M buffer, adapt, and innovate in response to external forces, particularly policy and funding influences (McBeath et al., 2014; Schmid, 2019). It is now harder for scholars to study the relationships between public policies and institutions on the one hand, and their community and human health consequences on the other hand, without including the study of organizations and their mediating roles (Dunne, Grady, & Weir, 2018; Krieger, 2001; Pierson, 2011). If "the drive-train of inequality runs from national institutions, to organizational structures, to the distribution of individual rewards" (Davis, 2017, p. 723), then a sensible path for the testing, refinement, and improvement of human service innovations runs through their organizational and societal context (Birken et al., 2017).

Second, research enhances understanding of how HSO&M influence policymaking through public and private advocacy (Mosley, 2020). For example, recent national initiatives to envision the future of social welfare include the Grand Challenges for Social Work led by the American Academy of Social Work and Social Welfare (AASWSW) (Fong, Lubben, & Barth, 2017) as well as the Council on Social Work Education (CSWE) Futures Task Force (Council on Social Work Education [CSWE], 2018). Each underscores the importance of transformational leaders and net-works of human service organizations in spurring social innovations in practices and programs, leading to changes in the social work profession and globally. The two initiatives reflect a rational approach to planning and policymaking, in which strategic visioning supports strategic planning, thereby informing policy advocacy and development (Bryson, 2018). Future scholarship on social welfare programs and policies will therefore involve research on HSO&M.

Third, research on HSO&M supports understanding of outcomes within organizations, and in particular, the effects of organizational structures and processes on individuals and groups. Issues concerning the consequences of human services and program activities within human service organiza-tions relate to questions of organizational culture and climate (Hemmelgarn & Glisson, 2018). Intra-organizationally, a clear goal is to examine whether human service staff and service users perceive their agency to be in alignment with their extrinsic motivations and intrinsic values and beliefs.

In sum, research on HSO&M responds to and/or anticipates the needs of practitioners and scholars. Such research concerns the space between thought and action – filling gaps between plans and actual practices as well as structuring effort in response to changing critical information (Argyris, 1993; Schön & Argyris, 1996). Research on HSO&M involves practice at all levels, ranging from the administration of clinical care in a single agency to industry-wide studies of social work education and workforce (e.g., Salsberg et al., 2019). Organizational and management questions should be asked relentlessly because they are so critical for learning and so difficult to answer comprehensively.

The contributions

The 10 commentaries comprising the special issue offer alternate visions of the practice and research context of HSO&M. The commentaries also propose future agendas to strengthen connections among social work micro practice and the macro practice domains of community practice, HSO&M practice, and policy practice.

The process

The special issue began with a June 2018 meeting of the journal editorial advisory board. In the meeting, we introduced the idea of a proposal for an invitational retreat during the 2019 annual conference of the Society for Social Work and Research (SSWR), in which scholars would be invited to contribute brief commentaries on the topic of "The Future of Human Service Organizational and Management Research". Responses to the idea referred to: the need to involve leaders of sister journals in social work macro practice as well as affiliated scholars; the campaign of the Special Commission to Advance Macro Practice to raise the profile of macro practice in regards to student enrollments and faculty educational curricula; and potential research and policy connections to be explored with the Grand Challenges for Social Work.

Fortified with these responses, we submitted an invitation in September 2018 to the editors of the other social work macro practice journals (*Journal of Community Practice, Journal of Policy Practice and Research, Journal of Technology in Human Services*) as well as select leading scholars of affiliated macro social work research domains (e.g., policy research, implementation science, health services research). Invitees were encouraged to contribute commentaries in response to two prompts: (a) What critical issue(s) face HSO&M researchers?; and (b) What HSO&M research (topics, questions, theories, methods) is most needed to address these critical issue(s)? Those who did not prepare a commentary were still encouraged to attend the workgroup meeting and contribute to dialogue.

Commentaries were shared with other commentators and attendees before the pre-conference retreat at SSWR on January 16, 2019. This was intended to give contributors time to refine their ideas in relation to the contributions of other commentators. Overall, the purpose of the retreat was to: (i) present diverse perspectives on the two questions reflecting contributors' theoretical and substantive backgrounds and current projects; and (ii) provide an opportunity to chart some contours of new practice and research developments, and exchange ideas, in a less-formal format (i.e., no PowerPoint presentations). After the retreat, commentators were encouraged to expand upon their thinking from the discussions. The commentaries were then peer-reviewed.

The commentaries

As presented, the 10 commentaries serve as distillations of intellectual and practical problem solving. Each commentator wrestles with self-selected practice puzzles while identifying possible solutions for the consideration of future scholar-researchers. The commentaries are active, novel, and challenging.

In "Pathways for Promoting Macro Practice in Social Work Education", Michael Austin identifies opportunities to integrate elements of macro practice curricula, and to re-center micro and macro practice in the milieu of the human service organization. Rather than having social work curricula silo macro practice into community, HSO&M, and policy practice courses and fieldwork, Austin argues for a trifocal integration of macro practice subdomains. In addition, through the linking of macro and micro practice courses with field experiences, he proposes that future practitioners should be encouraged to work more collaboratively using intersecting knowledge and skills, to support their continued growth and development as agency-based leaders. Austin also invites social work educators to use a design-based practice perspective to explore new curricular innovations that infuse an integrated approach to practice. He concludes by posing research questions concerning how, when, and why new instructional and practicum approaches contribute to successful micro-macro integration and student learning outcomes.

In "Implementation Science and Human Service Organizations Research: Opportunities and Challenges for Building on Complementary Strengths", Alicia Bunger and Rebecca Lengnick-Hall reflect upon the evolution of research on HSO&M in relation to the burgeoning field of implementation science. Our authors suggest that the perspectives share: a focus upon service quality outcomes in relation to the external environment of human service organizations; the search for relevant organizational and management frameworks to support program impact; and an emphasis in advancing research rigor. Bunger and Lengnick-Hall argue that through the alignment of common interests and the merging of distinct research methodologies and theoretical approaches, HSO&M researchers and implementation scientists should benefit from collaboration and ultimately work toward improving service delivery processes. They conclude with suggestions for scholar-researchers who are considering building conceptual and methodological bridges. Although their ideas pertain specifically to connections involving HSO&M research and implementation science, they can be applied sensibly to other applied scientific domains (e.g., HSO&M and prevention science).

Lauri Goldkind and John McNutt offer a compelling commentary in "We Could Be Unicorns: Human Service Leaders Moving from Managing Programs to Managing Information Ecosystems". They propose that new information and communication technologies (ICTs) and information ecologies are reshaping the roles of human service administrators, program managers, and line staff in delivering services. Our contributors thus distinguish between the management of traditional human service organizations versus the administration and leadership of information ecosystems. They argue that in response to evolving approaches to work and practice, educators and researchers should explore new theoretical frameworks (e.g., complexity science, collective intelligence) and practice frameworks emphasizing the management of peer networks and the support of parallel institutions. Goldkind and McNutt conclude by identifying needed practice skills for knowledge workers as well as new opportunities for curricular innovators and researchers.

Richard Hoefer begins his commentary on "Modest Challenges for the Fields of Human Service Administration and Social Policy Research and Practice" by cautioning that the Grand Challenges for Social Work appears to be an intellectual fad. Rather than jump to exploring the Grand Challenges, Hoefer argues that four Modest Challenges need to be addressed first: identifying competencies for social work administration and social policy; promoting engagement and inclusivity; improving human service pay and equity; and deciding whether to engage in advocacy. Each of these challenges is longstanding and is far from settled, largely because social workers have been unable to reconcile their often-competing dimensions. His commentary suggests that significant advocacy is needed to regularly re-envision macro practice competencies, promote engagement and inclusivity, and correct pay and equity imbalances. In concluding, Hoefer implies that local, sustained advocacy efforts in these domains may lead to more successful "moon shots" at a societal level.

In "Evaluating Behavioral and Organizational Outcomes of Leadership Development in Human Service Organizations", Karen Hopkins and Megan Meyer note that human service organizations often differentiate between practitioner knowledge acquisition and knowledge use, and between leadership development and organizational development. In contrast, our authors propose an integrated framework that involves leadership training to promote skill acquisition, followed by regular self-reflection and collaborative learning in program teams. Their framework is used to support the professional development of new leaders – particularly young women and persons of color who can receive vastly fewer opportunities for mentorship and collaboration. Hopkins and Meyer summarize their human service leadership and management training program involving the provision of a flexible, embedded-in-practice certificate program in tandem with an evaluation of the outcomes of leadership development and program performance. They conclude by suggesting the need to replicate, adapt, and further evaluate their program at the individual, collective/team, program, and organizational levels.

Bowen McBeath, Qing Tian, Bin Xu, and Jenifer Huang McBeath organize their commentary on "Human Service Organization-Environment Relationships in Relation to Environmental Justice: Old and New Approaches to Macro Practice and Research" via a basic claim: Human service organizations and managers pay insufficient attention to the built and natural environment and to environmental justice. In response, McBeath and colleagues affirm an environmental justice agenda for future macro practice, education, research, and theory. Drawing upon interdisciplinary literatures, the contributors locate challenges to environmentally just practice at the organizational and community levels – notably the lack of essential capacity to support service collaborations. They also ask whether environmental justice interventions in human service organizations can be transformative and sustainable. The authors conclude by reorienting HSO&M practitioners and researchers to questions of organization-environment relations, environmental justice, and supports for participatory, anti-oppressive practice.

In "The Practice and Science of Social Good: A New Framework to Guide Future Human Service Organizational and Management Research", Michalle Mor Barak introduces the "social good" movement, which she characterizes as including formal organizations, informal bodies, and actors seeking to benefit society through innovative change strategies that harness technology and collaborative ventures for positive social impact. Her concept of social good responds to multiple developments, including: progressive reactions to austerity and populism; theories of social capital, virtue, and justice; and practice in social entrepreneurship, macro social work, environmental justice, peace/nonviolence, and inclusion work. She introduces a social good framework for future HSO&M research that integrates the search for new theories, research questions, collaborations, measurement approaches, and technological applications. In her conclusion, Mor Barak reflects upon the historic roots of the social work profession while offering a vision of interorganizational, cross-sector macro practice partnerships.

Jennifer Mosley, Nicole Marwell, and Marci Ybarra locate their commentary "How the 'What Works' Movement Is Failing Human Service Organizations, and What Social Work Can Do to Fix It" in the ongoing struggle to use the science of social work to affirm the legitimacy of human services. Their provocative commentary highlights the unintended consequences of evidence-based interventions, tied to funding in particular, that require careful attention (if not strict adherence) to implementation despite contextual situations, compromised workforce education and training, and service inequities. Mosley, Marwell, and Ybarra remind us that not all forms of social service delivery can adequately incorporate EBPs and evidence-based policies, especially when dictated from disciplines outside of the social work sphere with less understanding of organizational factors and community dynamics. An important tenet of their commentary is the critical role of an advocacy-oriented organizational learning perspective for human service managers and workers to assess, adapt, and scale promising practices in order to better serve communities. They conclude by offering important research strategies to promote equity and service improvement in human service organizations and the social work profession.

In "De-Implementation of Evidence-Based Interventions: Implications for Organizational and Managerial Research", Rogerio Pinto and Sunggeun Park offer an essential premise: HSO&M practitioners may not know whether, when, and how to de-implement an EBP. De-implementing an EBP can take a toll on providers, community partners, and community members; yet research on promising practices for de-implementation of EBPs and for replacing interventions is largely nonexistent. Their commentary is particularly timely given that many human service organizations have struggled to effectively and efficiently implement EBPs, only to discover that these practices may not achieve the results intended, the interventions may cause harm, and larger contextual factors (i.e., political and economic pressures) within and beyond a program or organization may make the intervention irrelevant. Pinto and Park reflect upon their community-based research studies of the shifting terrain of evidence-based HIV preventive interventions in order to share key insights for HSO&M practitioners, researchers, and theorists. Their recommendation for practitioners and researchers to think through the consequences of any new intervention is valuable at all levels of practice.

Finally, Anna Maria Santiago and Richard Smith couch their commentary "What Can 'Big Data' Methods Offer Human Services Research on Organizations and Communities" in the perspective that while "big data" applications are increasingly being used to drive agency and community decision-making, human service professionals and researchers are often unable to articulate the varieties of big data and their consequences. Our contributors provide a rich overview of data science methodologies, offer examples of how current data science methods are used to respond to societal dilemmas, and identify specific practice and ethical concerns that relate to HSO&M. Santiago and Smith conclude by offering: a framework for interdisciplinary, intentional graduate education for social work students and human service professionals; and examples of possible research studies that describe and use data science methods for the testing and improvement of human service practices, programs, and policies. Their perspective implies that since data science is revolutionizing the world of human service work and the daily responsibilities of human service workers, the task at hand is to use data science research methodologies effectively and ethically.

Integrative themes regarding current challenges and proposed strategies

We now review themes concerning the challenges that commentators identify as well as the strategies that they propose. These themes concern: (1) increasing complexity facing the external and internal environment of practice; leading to (2) proposed approaches for managing complexity across levels of practice; resulting in (3) implications for the future of macro practice, research, and education. We develop each theme in turn.

Increasing complexity facing the environment of practice

The first theme relates to the fundamental complexity of the environment of practice. Although complexity is a characteristic of practice at all levels, some commentators suggest that complexity is increasing at an international level with national and local repercussions. Mor Barak refers to the volatility of recent economic trends and geopolitical concerns (e.g., immigration and refugee assistance) as driving nationalism and populism. Similarly, the commentary by McBeath and colleagues is situated in a VUCA (i.e., volatile, uncertain, complex, ambiguous) environment of climate change, natural and built disasters, and other socioecological hazards.

Other contributors propose that increasing complexity is affecting the immediate external environment of human service organizations. Mosley, Marwell, and Ybarra highlight the increased demands of public institutions (notably public funders and legislative bodies) being placed upon public and private human service providers. At the interorganizational level, Pinto and Park, and Bunger and Lengnick-Hall, identify challenges facing human service organizations in initiating and sustaining collaborative provider networks. And Santiago and Smith, and Goldkind and McNutt, refer to the challenges of integrating new technological developments (e.g., big data, ICTs) into existing human service systems. Finally, commentators allude to increasing societal and community needs, and increased concerns of diversity, equity, and inclusion, that are shaping the interorganizational and organizational milieu of human services.

Increasingly intense and uncertain extra-organizational forces have internal consequences within public and private human service organizations. Commentators generally note the difficulties associated with the delivery of high-need services while mitigating fiscal and management capacity challenges. They also describe ongoing workforce challenges involving the equitable retention and development of social service workers, particularly early career professionals and persons of color, amidst the demands and pressures of daily practice.

Is the pace of change accelerating for practitioners? Our commentators may think so. Goldkind and McNutt argue that the technological demands being placed upon human service workers are increasing exponentially. And Santiago and Smith explain that big data-driven decision-making can involve near real-time data reporting and visualization, particularly in European social welfare contexts. Other commentators imply that organizations are required to respond to new and ongoing demands in an uncertain climate, even though time is insufficient and HSO&M knowledge may be unavailable. For example, Hopkins and Meyer allude to the dependence of agency leaders upon just-in-time work procedures. Austin reminds us that macro practice faculty must compete for limited curricular shelf space and faculty supports amidst a possible overall decline in macro practice. And McBeath and colleagues raise the existential threat of climate change and industrial and natural disasters as a prelude to their commentary.

How should practitioners manage complexity?

The question thus becomes how future practitioners should manage complexity, and how to lead those who are responsible for its management. Commentators generally emphasize the importance of growing and strengthening reciprocal, trust-based partnerships to support collaborative problem solving and team learning. This conceptualization of practice involves attention to the perspectives of service users and community members in alliance with organizational learning approaches characterized by inclusive engagement with community agency partners. It can also foster design-based practice (as noted by Austin, Hopkins and Meyer, and Mor Barak), in which prototyping, design research, and market analysis spur the growth of new innovations. Such proposals offer an essential role for HSO&M research, but need not involve university-based researchers.

The paths proposed by the commentators are ambitious, and range from more settled and secure to rockier and more challenging. Some of the scenarios offered by our authors are embedded in existing organizational and institutional arrangements, and involve adaptations of current practices and programming (e.g., integrating macro practice more fully into existing social work courses). In contrast, other proposals are more in the form of visioning efforts. Mosley, Marwell, and Ybarra argue that a focus on organizational learning is an intermediate objective toward the goal of engaging in social reform to transform social structures. Hoefer notes that successful responses to his four Modest Challenges should pave the way for researchers and educators to address Grand

Challenges more effectively and ethically. McBeath and colleagues propose environmental justice initiatives that run the gamut from more bureaucratic to more community-based and anti-oppressive. Mor Barak envisions the creation of interdisciplinary social good marketplaces that involve collaborative ventures across sectors and countries for social impact. And Goldkind and McNutt imagine the development of information ecosystems as well as the growth of alternative social institutions.

Implicit in the commentaries is the idea of leadership as local and relational, and as involving community, organizational, and policy practice. Contributors also reaffirm the importance of "pressing pause" by incorporating diverse types of knowledge before charting a course of action. The concept of pressing pause in light of new perspectives is exemplified by the commentaries focused upon EBP implementation:

- Bunger and Lengnick-Hall invite researchers to collaborate with community partners to look under the proverbial hood of EBPs in order to identify their active mechanisms of change.
- Mosley, Marwell, and Ybarra ask practitioners, researchers, and policymakers whether EBPs have unintended consequences and collateral effects (e.g., the loss of local knowledge and community-based learning).
- Pinto and Park imply that the space between de-implementation of existing EBPs and the start of new interventions involves opportunities for community-based engagement and leadership.

Pressing pause is thus a hallmark of effective management and leadership in increasingly complex circumstances. The concept is aligned with the theory of collective intelligence alluded to by Goldkind and McNutt, and is a core principle of organizational learning (Argyris, 1993; Schön & Argyris, 1996). It is a sensible strategy for practitioners, educators, and researchers who are asked to follow poorly-marked paths, or who are interested in building new trails.

Implications for the future of macro practice, research, and education

The commentaries suggest some domains of inquiry regarding the future of macro research and education vis-à-vis macro practice. The first concerns the importance of assessing the impacts of new technologies in the helping professions. Macro practitioners are not exempt from training and supporting social workers and related professionals to have familiarity (if not facility) with big data in complex knowledge economies. The concerns raised by our contributors are echoed by the Grand Challenges for Social Work and the CSWE Futures Task Force. We therefore wonder how macro practitioners can stay abreast of technological opportunities while addressing workforce and policy-program concerns. In addition, Hasenfeld (2010) reminded us that human service technologies: are indeterminate and involve ethical considerations; can involve competition and collaboration for essential resources (e.g., funding) and legitimacy; and resultantly involve politics, gender, and culture. Researchers and educators therefore have an opportunity to investigate the economic, political, and social ramifications of new technologies.

The second domain relates to global and local arenas for social and environmental justice practice. The commentaries serve as examples of: broader exploration of the roles of macro practitioners in relation to capital flows, international relations, and identity politics; and deeper investigation of place-based concerns involving the built and natural environment that reflect the adage ascribed to former U.S. Speaker of the House of Representatives Tip O'Neill that "all politics is local" (Austin, 2018, p. 599). Their braided analysis expands traditional notions of human behavior in the social environment, policy and program development and analysis, and macro practice (notably advocacy). How do cross-sector partnerships, collaborations, and networks get formed? Which leaders and organizations are responsible and accountable for collective goods? How do we effectively measure the processes and impacts of change efforts in global and local arenas? We thus see opportunities for future research and education concerning social and environmental justice practice in relation to organization-environment analysis as well as community and stakeholder theory development.

The third domain involves organizational learning to support service delivery and community benefits. At the service delivery level, contributors are examining the constellation of factors involved in EBPs, implementation science and policy/program implementation, and contextual influences. All of these factors are important; yet a critical lens is needed to decipher which are essential. At the programmatic and organizational levels, commentators are situating service outcomes and results in relation to questions of what works, the nature of evidence, and accountability to partners and funders. At a basic level, macro research and education are needed to ensure that action research studies result in practical, accessible data from the perspectives of diverse partners. Finally, at the community leadership and workforce level, we see opportunities to use practical research and training to support and evaluate leadership development and the growth of local social enterprises.

The fourth domain is specific to professional education in social work, allied health professions (e.g., public health, nursing), and public and nonprofit management. What should we realistically be teaching students to demonstrate, to assess them as competent and competitive human service professionals? Across the commentaries, the following learning capacities are heralded as necessary:

- The integration of community, organizational and leadership, and policy practice in combination with micro practice.
- Deeper and more local as well as broader and more global understanding of human behavior in relation to the social environment of practice and theory.
- ICTs and data science technologies in relation to service technologies (including EBPs and implementation science) at multiple levels of practice.
- Access to and appropriate use of diverse forms of knowledge for research-practice advocacy partnerships and relational learning.

We wonder whether any professional curriculum is sufficiently organized to prepare students for these practice domains.

A final issue concerns whether schools of social work have sufficient institutional resources to connect micro, meso, and macro practice with research. This issue is not new. Whittaker (2002) noted that as the 1970s- and 1980s-era social R&D models were replaced by early EBP frameworks in the 1990s, leading schools, national associations, governmental bodies, and foundations were needed to reduce the balkanization of social work research, education, and practice. Looking to the future, our commentators argue that university leaders and professional associations (e.g., AASWSW, CSWE, SSWR) are still unprepared to support practical knowledge, scientific research, and educational programming across levels of practice. Indeed, Hoefer notes that we struggle to address basic challenges at a local level, let alone the Grand Challenges at national and international levels. We therefore pose a simple question: If connections between levels of practice, and between practice and research, are variable at best at top U.S. schools of social work, then what is the prognosis for non-R1 schools and departments?

Reflection on the future of human service organizational and management research

Our introduction to the special issue illuminates that which is essential-yet-hidden, often in plain view. Organizational and managerial work is quintessentially boundary spanning labor – i.e., difficult to do well and often collectively regarded as essential only when it is absent. Research centered in HSO&M bridges the gap between knowing and doing within organizations and across them. As described by our contributors, such research is regularly situated in the perspectives of service users and community members, attentive to policy demands amidst practice dilemmas, and thus predominantly local and relational. HSO&M research is needed to transition from community-based learning to the development and enhancement of innovative, anti-bureaucratic practices, programs, and policies. It is also needed to organize advocacy within and beyond human service systems. Finally, research on HSO&M is needed to implement and evaluate strategic responses to Grand Challenges.

Yet our commentators imply that the opportunities presented to HSO&M researchers come with corresponding external challenges, notably insufficient resources for applied research. Another challenge involves the question of the time needed for HSO&M researchers to do important work vs. the complexity of the tasks at hand. A futurist sees possibilities; our commentators instead reflect upon real-world probabilities that have been occurring over decades, and that are expected to accelerate. It has been argued that all major change is intergenerational. If this is so, then one may be concerned that research on HSO&M is increasingly important because the time needed to connect planning to action is increasingly limited.

Other challenges are internal to who we are and what we do as HSO&M researchers. Notably, what should organizational and management researchers make of the messy boundaries between micro and macro practice, and between social work and sister professions and disciplines? One can argue that organizational and management research provides the essential connective tissues between frontline services research and research on their historical-institutional, policy, and civic contexts. Yet a counterargument is that organizational and management research is neither fish nor fowl – i.e., not properly rooted in frontline methodologies and theories, and not adequately situated in relation to the policy sciences and the increasingly methodologically and theoretically sophisticated literatures of public and nonprofit management.

It is not the aim of this special issue to call for a rapprochement between practice, theory, and methodology across levels of analysis. Our perspective, in contrast, is that HSO&M research should involve the use of social and behavioral science methodologies and available theoretical tools to support the needs of human service organizations and managers according to their sense of time. This may suggest that HSO&M researchers should remain eclectic in conceptualizing and operationalizing practice, research, and theory. However, we believe there are real opportunities for specialization in HSO&M research subdomains, including the five we summarized above. Although our commentators have offered many examples in response, examples are often not exemplary. A future question is therefore how HSO&M can be more methodologically rigorous, accessible to practice and timely, and relevant to theory building and refinement. And we see the need for future HSO&M researchers who can resolve the trilemma of having excellent research methods, careful theorizing, and rich and rapid connections to practice.

We conclude by reaffirming the importance of this journal as a place to bridge HSO&M research and practice. As reflected in the 10 commentaries of the special issue, the contributors are challenging us to press pause: to avoid locked-in syndromes; to step out of our comfort zones; and to explore new terrains by posing complex questions. Finally, our contributors are arguing for possible resolutions to longstanding problems and new challenges and opportunities in human service organizational and management practice, research, and education.

Disclosure statement

No potential conflict of interest was reported by the authors.

References

Adedoyin, A. C., Miller, M., Jackson, M. S., Dodor, B., & Hall, K. (2016). Faculty experiences of merger and organizational change in a social work program. *Journal of Evidence-Informed Social Work*, 13, 87–98. doi:10.1080/15433714.2014.997094

Argyris, C. (1993). *Knowledge for action: A guide to overcoming barriers to organizational change*. San Francisco, CA: Jossey-Bass.

Austin, M. J. (2018). Social work management practice, 1917–2017: A history to inform the future. *Social Service Review*, 92, 548–616. doi:10.1086/701278

Birken, S. A., Bunger, A. C., Powell, B. J., Turner, K., Clary, A. S., Klaman, S. L., … Chatham, J. R. S. (2017). Organizational theory for dissemination and implementation research. *Implementation Science*, 12, 62. doi:10.1186/s13012-017-0592-x

Bryson, J. M. (2018). *Strategic planning for public and nonprofit organizations: A guide to strengthening and sustaining organizational achievement*. New York, NY: Wiley.

Call, C. R., Owens, L. W., & Vincent, N. J. (2013). Leadership in social work education: Sustaining collaboration and mission. *Advances in Social Work, 14,* 594–612. doi:10.18060/3502

Council on Social Work Education. (2018, April). *Envisioning the future of social work* (Report of the CSWE Futures Task Force). Washington, DC: Author.

Davis, G. F. (2017). How organizations create income inequality. In R. Greenwood, C. Oliver, T. B. Lawrence, & R. E. Meyer (Eds.), *The Sage handbook of organizational institutionalism* (2nd ed., pp. 722–737). Thousand Oaks, CA: Sage.

Dunne, S., Grady, J., & Weir, K. (2018). Organization studies of inequality, with and beyond Piketty. *Organization, 25,* 165–185. doi:10.1177/1350508417714535

Fong, R., Lubben, J., & Barth, R. P. (Eds.). (2017). *Grand challenges for social work and society.* New York, NY: Oxford University Press.

Hasenfeld, Y. (1983). *Human service organizations.* Englewood Cliffs, NJ: Prentice-Hall.

Hasenfeld, Y. (2010). The attributes of human service organizations. In Y. Hasenfeld (Ed.), *Human services as complex organizations* (pp. 9–32). Thousand Oaks, CA: Sage.

Hemmelgarn, A. L., & Glisson, C. (2018). *Building cultures and climates for effective human services: Understanding and improving organizational social contexts with the ARC model.* New York, NY: Oxford University Press.

Krieger, N. (2001). Theories for social epidemiology in the 21st century: An ecosocial perspective. *International Journal of Epidemiology, 30,* 668–677. doi:10.1093/ije/30.4.668

Lewis, H. (1977). The future role of the social service administrator. *Administration in Social Work, 1,* 115–122. doi:10.1300/J147v01n02_01

McBeath, B., Collins-Camargo, C., Chuang, E., Wells, R., Bunger, A. C., & Jolles, M. P. (2014). New directions for research on the organizational and institutional context of child welfare agencies: Introduction to the symposium on "the organizational and managerial context of private child welfare agencies". *Children and Youth Services Review, 38,* 83–92. doi:10.1016/j.childyouth.2014.01.014

Menefee, D. (2009). What human services managers do and why they do it. In R. J. Patti (Ed.), *The handbook of human services management* (pp. 101–116). Thousand Oaks, CA: Sage.

Mosley, J. E. (2020). Social service nonprofits: Navigating conflicting demands. In W. W. Powell & P. Bromley (Eds.), *The nonprofit sector: A research handbook.* Palo Alto, CA: Stanford University Press.

Patti, R. J. (2009). Management in the human services. In R. J. Patti (Ed.), *The handbook of human services management* (pp. 3–27). Thousand Oaks, CA: Sage.

Pierson, P. (2011). *Politics in time: History, institutions, and social analysis.* New York, NY: Princeton University Press.

Salsberg, E., Quigley, L., Richwine, C., Sliwa, S., Acquaviva, K., & Wyche, K. (2019, April). *From social work education to social work practice: Results of the survey of 2018 social work graduates* (A report to the Council on Social Work Education and National Workforce Steering Initiative). Alexandria, VA: The George Washington University Health Workforce Institute.

Schmid, H. (2019). Rethinking organizational reforms in human service organizations: Lessons, dilemmas, and insights. *Human Service Organizations: Management, Leadership, & Governance, 43,* 54–66.

Schön, D., & Argyris, C. (1996). *Organizational learning II: Theory, method and practice.* Reading, UK: Addison Wesley.

Slavin, S. (1977). Editorial. *Administration in Social Work, 1,* 1–2.

Whittaker, J. K. (2002). The practice-research nexus in social work: Problems and prospects. *Social Service Review, 76,* 686–694. doi:10.1086/343000

Pathways for Promoting Macro Practice in Social Work Education: A Commentary

Michael J. Austin

ABSTRACT

As we approach the third decade of the twenty-first century, it is time to move beyond the wake-up call provided by the 2013 Rothman Report on the future of macro practice and its perceived decline. While most of the report's recommendations focused on the external environment related to recognition by national social work organizations and future enrollment targets (20% macro for entering MSW students), it is now timely to look internally to address our own issues. Faculty need to step back to assess their own capacities to integrate macro practice curriculum content, given the contracting "shelf space" of course offerings. This commentary explores three pathways to macro practice: 1) integrating community, management, and policy practice curricula, 2) re-positioning macro practice in the advanced practice curricula, and 3) revisiting the relationship between micro and macro practice related to the CSWE practice competencies. The commentary concludes with a future research agenda.

Overview

Macro practice has a rich and storied history in social work practice and education over the past 100 years (Austin, 2018; Gutierrez & Gant, 2018; Jansson, 2014). In this commentary, macro practice refers to the educational programs and career paths that include community practice, management practice, and policy practice. The parallel evolution of these three domains of macro practice over the past century informs their respective development as well as their impact on direct practice, the largest arena of social work practice. Their inter-relationships are explored in this commentary through the use of three pathways for promoting macro practice. The first pathway features *integrating elements of macro practice* and the second pathway *locates macro practice within the curriculum space of advanced social work practice*. And the third pathway is based on the assumption that *elements of macro practice are built into the curriculum of the foundation of social work practice* where it is possible to build bridges between micro and macro practice. The commentary also draws upon the macro practice knowledge base that is found, in part, in the three major macro practice journals of the profession (*Human Service Organizations*, founded in 1977; *Journal of Community Practice*, founded in 1992; *Journal of Policy Practice*, founded in 2001).

Urgency of this commentary

For many years, the marketplace for attracting social workers to the arena of macro practice has been the human services sector. Applicants to macro practice social work programs were often staff members of nonprofit human service organizations where they learned about social work when working in schools, hospitals, youth organizations, senior centers, Peace Corp and Americorp volunteers, and others. While they may have begun their careers in the human service providing direct services to clients, many became intrigued with organizational roles related to inter-agency planning, program management, and policy advocacy. These experiences led them to discover that there were social work graduate programs that included specializations in one or more domains of macro practice.

At the same time, competition in the marketplace has increased dramatically with the proliferation of undergraduate and graduate programs in nonprofit management, public administration, and public policy. While many of the prospective applicants may have interest in leading and managing human service organizations, they are usually unaware of this career option when it is buried in the curriculum of a school of social work. In a parallel development, there are those disenchanted with the corporate life as well as undergraduate social science majors looking to make a difference in the lives of others.

While the enrollments in the area of macro social work practice have grown in a few large (often public) universities, they have declined or disappeared in other universities where the demand (from students and agencies) to educate direct service practitioners continues to expand. By the beginning of the twenty-first century, there was a growing concern about the reductions in macro practice offerings in schools of social work that led to a "wake-up call" in the form of the 2013 Rothman Report commissioned by ACOSA as highlighted in Figure 1.

The report was built upon a literature review and faculty survey. The literature review captured the following highlights: 1) macro practice has become "a marginalized subfield in social work" (Fisher and

Faculty Issues	Curriculum Issues
• Many faculty in schools of social work lack interest in or oppose macro courses and programs • Little or no hiring of macro faculty • Some deans/directors do not value the macro curriculum or provide adequate resources to support it • In research-oriented schools, there is an overemphasis on securing large federal clinical/population research grants that downplay macro research perspectives	• The primary structure of the vast majority of school's curriculum is clinical • Licensure requires many micro courses and leads to little attention to macro content • Macro courses are neglected or marginalized by disinterest in course content or those teaching the courses • There is limited integration of macro with micro in the curriculum (despite decades of attention to generalist practice) • Faculty do not encourage students to take macro courses or value the macro practice perspective • In some schools, macro practice field placements are lacking or problematic

Student Issues
• General lack of interest among clinical students in macro practice

Figure 1. Education for macro practice (2013 Rothman report)*.
*Rothman (2013). *Education for macro intervention: A survey of problems and prospects*. Los Angeles: University of California, Los Angeles (https://www.acosa.org/joomla/pdf/RothmanReportRevisedJune2013.pdf).

Corciullo, 2011, p. 359), 2) as of 2011, MSW student enrollment in macro areas reached 8.8% (management or administration, 2.4%; community planning/organization, 2.1%; combined community planning and management administration, 2.7%; social policy, 1%; combined social policy and program evaluation, 0.6%), 3) according to the NASW Center for Workforce Studies, 14% of social workers identify macro as their practice focus (Whitaker & Arrington, 2008), 4) there is a considerable shortage of social work practitioners with the full range of knowledge, skills, and experience needed to tackle immense challenges facing low-income neighborhoods (Mott, 2008), and 5) in addition to the somewhat random nature of on-the-job training, the primary vehicles for developing entry-level macro practice social work competencies for the profession are located in schools of social work.

The ACOSA Report led to the publication of the Macro Practice Guide (CSWE, 2018) for social work educators by the Council on Social Work Education. At the same time, the Network for Social Work Managers (2018) revised its guide to *Human Services Management Competencies*. By 2019, the workforce study of the Council on Social Work Education (2019) reported that recent graduates had selected the following areas of specialization: direct practice (81.5%) and macro practice that included community organizing, policy advocacy, and indirect management practice (17.2%). It seems that the national goal of 20% macro practice may be within reach.

The underlying theme of this commentary includes the need to balance a sense of urgency with a sense of calm about addressing the future of social work macro practice on campus and in the community. Even though a few schools of social work possess a strong investment in macro practice in terms of student and faculty resources, macro practice in general is competing for limited social work curriculum space and faculty support. In essence, the lessons from the past suggest a need for more urgency than calm when it comes to the future of social work macro practice. The past is briefly captured in the detour that follows.

Reflecting upon teaching macro practice

As a newly-minted assistant professor nearly 50 years ago (1970) with an MSW in community organizing and administration and a PhD in organizational research, I was confronted with my first teaching challenge; namely, specifying course content and identifying relevant literature. I was hired to start-up the macro practice component of a predominantly direct service or casework school. With little guidance from available course outlines and the limited literature (Kahn, 1969; Rothman & Jones, 1971; Schatz, 1970), I found myself deeply influenced by my MSW experience with my mentor, Ralph Kramer and his social work background in community organizing and social planning (Kramer & Specht, 1969). While most of the literature reflected the nonprofit sector, my practice experience related primarily to federal government programs (War on Poverty and Community Mental Health) which proved to be very helpful since I landed in a school located in a state capitol with very few student fieldwork placement opportunities except in state government human service agencies.

During my first few years of teaching, the community practice literature grew exponentially (Note 1). By the late 1970s and early 1980s, the management practice literature also grew significantly (Note 2). By the 1980s, a new journal had emerged (*Administration in Social Work*, 1977 and later changed to *Human Service Organizations* in 2012) and macro faculty were searching for peer support and information exchange at annual CSWE meetings when they formed a section of the Council on Social Work Education in 1987 known as ACOSA (Association for Community Organizing and Social Administration).

These developments also led to the founding of the *Journal on Community Practice* in 1992 and the *Journal of Policy Practice* in 2001. While the teaching of macro practice continued to followed the separate tracks institutionalized by the three different journals, there were beginning efforts to lay the macro practice groundwork for integrating the three areas of community, management and policy practice (Austin, 1986). Many of these efforts took the form of "advanced social work practice" that sought to integrate micro and macro practice in order to supplement the education of students focused on direct practice. Some of the leadership in this area of curriculum development came from faculty teaching in undergraduate BSW programs who were interested in providing a more comprehensive approach to social work practice. This theme is explored later in this commentary.

Pathway #1: integrating elements of macro practice

By "fast forwarding" from a brief history to the twenty-first century, new challenges emerged in the search for the theoretical foundations for macro practice. Given the long history of providing course content in the area of human behavior in the social environment (HBSE), it became increasingly clear that more attention was being devoted to understanding human behavior within a micro practice context and less attention to the social environment within a macro practice context. The major exception to this perspective was the long-standing commitment in social work education to the teaching of social policy so that practitioners across the micro-mezzo-macro practice spectrum could engage in policy-informed practice.

Trifocal theory perspective for macro practice

Given that the social environment is a critical domain for macro practice, new efforts emerged to define this arena (Taylor, Austin, & Mulroy, 2004a, 2004b). Similar to the long European tradition of theory-informed practice, there was a need to move from theory familiarity that is most common in the social sciences (resource dependency theory, political economy theory, critical race theory, etc.) to a set of key concepts derived from community, organizational, and group theory (Mulroy & Austin, 2004). This body of theory is drawn from a considerable knowledge base constructed by Hasenfeld (1983), Fellin (2001), and Levi (2018) and provides a foundation for theory-informed macro practice as noted in Figure 2.

A set of concepts derived from the contributions of social work and related scholars were selected to provide macro practitioners with the tools to engage in assessing the dynamics of communities, groups, and organizations through the use of a trifocal perspective. The key concepts included in the assessment "tool box" include the structure and process of a group, community, or organization where the trifocal perspective also includes other concepts to assess: stages of development, power and leadership, systems of exchange, conflict and change, integrating mechanisms, diversity, and practitioner–environment interactions as noted in Figure 3 (Mulroy & Austin, 2004).

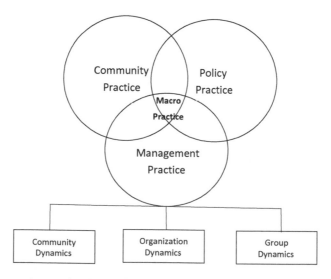

Figure 2. Balancing macro practice on a foundation of theories about human behavior and the social environment.

- Structure and Processes: *Structure* refers to the arrangement and mutual relationships of the constituent parts of a community, organization or group while *process* is defined as a continuous series of actions, events or changes that are directed toward some goal and/or performed in a specific manner in the community, organization or group.

- Stages of Development: Refers to the location of the community, group, or organization along a continuum of time and evolution that relates to stability over time or its changing nature (improving or declining).

- Systems of Exchange: Mechanisms designed to foster mutual support in a social environment that recognizes the central role of "self-interest" in communities, organizations, and groups within the context of giving and receiving.

- Intersectionality of diverse populations: Refers to differences between individuals and groups with respect to social identities and distinctive characteristics based on gender, race, sexual orientation, culture, age, ability, social class, and religion within a context of commonalities as well as shared respect, goals and concerns.

- Power and Leadership: *Power* is defined as the capacity to influence others as well as the ability to exercise authority and control. *Leadership* involves the effective use of power in terms of influencing and guiding others.

- Conflict and Change: *Conflict* is defined as a struggle between different perspectives (where positive conflict can promote understanding and integration while negative conflict can lead to alienation and fragmentation) and *change* is defined as making something different that sometimes emerges out of conflict.

- Integrating Mechanisms: Refers to networks of relationships that hold communities, groups and organizations together in the form of institutionalized processes or procedures used to monitor and provide feedback on their health and well-being.

- Practitioner-environment Interaction: Represents the relationships between the social environment (community, group and organization) and self-reflective practice of practitioners where the reciprocal interaction between neighborhood residents (community) and practitioners (influence each other), peers in a group (influence each other), and supervisors and supervisees in organizations (influence each other).

Figure 3. Core concepts as tools for assessing the dynamics of communities, groups, and organizations*.
*Mulroy and Austin (2004). Toward a comprehensive framework for understanding the social environment: In search of theory for practice. *Journal of Human Behavior and the Social Environment*, 10(3), 25–59.

While the trifocal perspective for assessing the dynamics of communities, groups, and organizations relates to theory-informed practice, it can serve as a foundation for macro practice community program design and needs assessment, managing program implementation, and policy practice related to coalition-building and advocacy. In addition to supporting theory-informed practice, the trifocal framework can also be used to structure the integration of core macro practice skills drawn from the three practice domains in the form of a trifocal intervention perspective. An integrated definition of macro practice features *managing* interventions in the community (formerly community practice) (Weil, 2005), *organizing* the community of internal and external stakeholders, inside and outside human service organizations (formerly management practice) (Menefee, 2009), and *building coalition-based advocacy* related to developing and implementing new policies (formerly policy practice) (Donaldson, 2008).

As Weil (2005) notes, community practice encompasses four central skills: 1) enabling and empowering people to work together to change their lives and environment, 2) organizing communities of interest, 3) designing, coordinating, and changing programs and services that are appropriate for different communities, and 4) developing and sustaining groups and coalitions engaged in social, economic, and political action. These processes are all relevant to that aspect of macro practice that features managing interventions in the community. In a parallel process, the management aspects of macro practice relate to organizing the community of internal and external stakeholders, inside and outside human service organizations and include three major functions: 1) leadership roles (boundary-spanner, innovator, organizer, team builder), 2) teamwork (communicator, supervisor, advocate, facilitator), and 3) analytics (resource manager, evaluator, policy analyst) (Menefee, 2009). And finally, the policy practice dimensions of macro practice focus on coalition-based advocacy related to developing and implementing new policies. The key functions in this area include: 1) monitoring the social and policy context of services to promote advocacy, 2) utilizing the knowledge of constituents (expertise of experience) for advocacy, 3) utilizing knowledge of program staff (expertise of training/experience), 4) working in coalitions to engage in advocacy and provide political cover, and 5) maintaining focus on an area of expertise for greatest impact (Donaldson, 2008).

Within this context, macro practitioners are able to function effectively within all three contexts; namely, community, organizational, and policy advocacy. The cross-domain skills are noted in Figure 4 and reflect the following: 1) leading by empowering others, 2) organizing for teamwork, and 3) planning by capturing information and expertise. With these skill sets in mind, it should be possible to move away from traditionally segregated macro practice content into more cross-cutting knowledge and skill dissemination using the traditional containers of semesters or quarters. This approach also suggests that seminars used to support fieldwork could also be structured around these practice themes. These three re-conceptualized practice skill-sets also allow for more customization with regard to student learning projects and faculty efforts to use simulations and other forms of experiential learning to reinforce these integrated macro practice domains.

Pathway #2: the macro practice dimensions of advanced social work practice

While the first pathway addressed those individuals investing in a career in macro practice, the second pathway addresses those focused on providing direct services to individuals, families, and groups. However, this pathway has a history of considerable debate (Hernandez, 2008). The concept of advanced practice emerged in the 1980s in response to the increased interest in defining the foundation of practice for both BSW and MSW consideration. Advanced practice was not defined by CSWE and it was left to each school to develop its own configuration. For some, it represented specialized fields of practice like children and families, aging, behavioral, health, housing, and other fields. For others, advanced practice related specifically to practice as in clinical practice, management practice, community practice, policy practice and other areas of practice. And finally for those schools without sufficient student interest or faculty expertise, the third option was a mix of micro and macro practice. It is this third option that is the focus of this section. It relies heavily on the interests and expertise of the faculty when it comes to defining advanced social work practice; namely, those with strong clinical expertise may seek to complement their backgrounds with expertise in the mezzo and macro areas of practice in an effort to create a balance between micro, mezzo, and macro course content.

Within this context of limited curricular shelf space, textbooks have been developed to address the role that macro practice can play in the daily routines of micro practitioners. For example, in order to make community organizing practice more accessible, Hardina (2013) focuses on the interpersonal skills needed for community organizing practice. These skills include the domains of pre-engagement, engagement, and post-engagement along with a focus on the interpersonal skills related to advocacy, community-building, staff supervision, and human rights advocacy. Similarly with other colleagues (Hardina,

I.   Leading by empowering others

- Organizational leadership roles (boundary-spanner, innovator, organizer, team builder) (MP)
- Community development processes (e.g. enabling and empowering people to work in united ways to change their lives and environment) (CP)
- Taking action for progressive change (e.g. developing and sustaining groups and coalitions engaged in social, economic, and political action) (CP)
- Policy practice of monitoring the social and policy context of services to promote advocacy (PP)
- Maintaining policy focus on an area of expertise for greatest impact (PP)

II.   Organizing for teamwork

- Organizational teamwork (communicator, supervisor, advocate, facilitator) (MP)
- Organizing (e.g. organizing communities of interest) (CP)
- Working in coalitions to engage in advocacy and provide political cover (PP)
- Ensuring full support by organizational/community leadership (staff, board & elected officials) (PP)

III.   Planning by capturing information and expertise

- Planning (e.g. designing, coordinating, and changing programs and services that are appropriate for different communities) (CP)
- Analyzing data to inform decision-making (managing financial and human resources, managing information systems, evaluation policy implementation and development) (MP)
- Utilizing the knowledge of constituents (expertise of experience) for advocacy (PP)
- Utilizing the knowledge of program staff (expertise of training/experience) (PP)

Figure 4. Integrating community, management and policy practice skills*.
*Based on community practice (CP) in the form of managing interventions in the community (Weil, 2005), management practice (MP) in the form of organizing the community of internal and external stakeholders, inside and outside human service organizations (Menefee, 2009), and policy practice (PP) in the form of coalition-based advocacy related to developing and implementing new policies (Donaldson, 2008).

Middleton, Montana, & Simpson, 2006), Hardina elaborates upon the management skills needed to empower human service organizations. These skills include managing empowerment-oriented social service agencies related to increasing consumer access and high-quality service programs, promoting organizational leadership, empowering staff, enhancing teamwork, engaging in policy practice, securing funding, evaluating services and programs, and promoting inter-agency relations. In a similar fashion, Netting, Kettner, McMurtry, and Thomas (2017) feature all three aspects of macro practice when the address community, management, and policy practice. In contrast, Reisch (2018) presents a more integrated approach of the major macro methods (e.g. community needs assessment, program development, working with groups, advocacy and media relations) and the theories that inform macro practice (e.g. organization–society relations, power and leadership, and the dynamics of conflict and change) as illustrated in Figure 5.

- Macro Practice in a Multicultural Society

- Theories Underlying Macro Social Work Practice in a Multicultural Society

- Human Service Organizations in a Multicultural Society

- Creating a Diverse Organizational Culture

- The External Environment of Macro Social Work Practice

- Power and Leadership in Multicultural Organizations and Communities

- Working With Diverse Groups in Macro Social Work Practice

- Identifying and Resolving Ethical Dilemmas in Macro Social Work Practice

- Defining "Community" and Assessing its Needs and Assets

- Engaging With and Intervening in Multicultural

- Advocating for Policy Change in the Legislative Arena

- Using Media as a Tool of Community, Organizational, and Social Change

- Advocacy in the Judicial, Executive, and Electoral Arenas

- Promoting Change and Dealing With Conflict in Multicultural Organizations

Figure 5. Dimensions of macro practice social work*.
*Reisch (2018). Macro practice social work: Working for change in a multi-cultural society. San Diego, CA: Cognella Academic Publishing.

Given that micro practice emphasizes the delivery of services to individuals and families, there is often little curricular space to address group work skills, except possibly the area of group therapy in an advanced clinical practice curriculum. Therefore, task groups which are essential for the conduct of organizational functioning (e.g. supervision, training, inter-disciplinary case conference, inter-agency service coordination) can also receive attention when balancing micro, mezzo, and macro content in an advanced practice curriculum (Toseland & Rivas, 2017). And finally, the third aspect of macro practice (beyond community and management) relates to policy practice that includes attention to advocacy and the empowerment of service users and citizens; namely, understanding politics, planning advocacy, and doing advocacy while also promoting citizen participation (VeneKlasen & Miller, 2007). This area of the curriculum has implications for the advocacy role of direct service practitioners (administrative, legal, community, and legislative) (Ezell, 2001) as well as managing the advocacy component of human service organizations (Kimberlin, 2010).

Given the challenges facing micro practitioners emerging from the demands and pressures of daily practice, it can be difficult to keep a focus on the mezzo and macro aspects of advanced generalist practice. In an effort to identify some of the core macro skills relevant to micro practice on an ongoing basis, several possibilities seem relevant. First, daily micro and macro practice often involves managing up, out and down (Austin, 1981, 1988, 2002) when it comes to addressing the needs of one's supervisor when managing up, addressing the needs of your colleagues inside and outside the agency when managing out, and addressing the needs of staff or volunteers when managing down. Each of these skill areas call for management skills when engaging others. Second, a great deal of the work carried out by micro and macro practitioners calls for teamwork and the group work skills needed to foster participation, demonstrate and recruit leadership, and manage differences related to diversity, conflict, and difficult conversations (Levi, 2018; Stone, Patton,

& Heen, 1999). Group work practice was a central ingredient in social work education in the twentieth century but has lost considerable curriculum support and faculty expertise in the twenty-first century. Agency-based fieldwork instructors are now in the primary role of educating the future generation by modeling and explaining group work skills but it is not clear that they have agreed to assume this role.

The third area of advanced social work practice relates to the role of community practice and how it is incorporated into effective clinical practice (Austin, Coombs, & Barr, 2005; Smale, 1995). In this context, community refers to the neighborhood location of the clients being served so that the impact of the social environment can be included in the assessment of human behavior. For example, if all the clients in an existing caseload were located with a dot on a neighborhood map, how familiar is the service provider with the changing conditions of those neighborhoods? Beyond the geographic community, attention can also be paid to the functional community with respect to engaging in inter-disciplinary case conferences (inside and outside the agency), inter-agency task forces (e.g. coordinating referrals and developing joint grant proposals for service expansion/redirection, assessing community impact of services provided). Another aspect of the community component of advanced social work practice relates to the skills called for in participatory action research designed to capture changing client populations needs and using findings to advocate for systems change that expands the micro practice role to include becoming a change agent. In essence, incorporating community practice skills into micro practice involves the similar skills used in micro practice (e.g. providing guidance and leadership, managing time, working with others, continuously defining purpose and outcomes, and making effective use of self).

Pathway #3: building bridges between micro and macro practice

Practitioners engaged in direct micro practice and those engaged in macro practice share several commonalities in addition to the social work values and ethics. First, they share a common workplace when it comes to responding to changing community needs and changing social policies. Second, both forms of practice share a common set of skills (Austin, Anthony, Knee, & Mathias, 2016). And third, micro and macro practice complement each other in ways that make the wholeness of their parts stronger than operating separately. Each of these shared characteristics is described in this section.

Sharing a common workplace

As noted by Gibelman and Furman (2008), the successful navigation of human service organizations (including nonprofit, public, and for-profit) requires both knowledge and skill. The knowledge areas include an understanding of the organization's history, mission, service programs, and rules and procedures. It is equally important to know how the organization functions as an open system that evolves and changes in response internally to those working with service users and externally to those partners engaged in coordination, service evaluation, and financial accountability. The functioning of the organization also involves the exercise of power as reflected in the role of the board of directors and executive director of a nonprofit and the role of elected officials in the hiring of the organization's director and monitoring performance. The staff at all levels of the agency need to understand the formal and informal organization chart comprised the various organizational leaders. Supervisors of practitioners play a key role by linking the concerns of staff with the concerns of top management. With a strong orientation to service accountability, supervisors carry out the three functions of implementing administrative policies and procedures (including personnel policies related to staff performance reviews and financial policies related to service program evaluations and quality assurance programs), supporting the changing needs of staff support, and promoting staff through ongoing education (Austin, 1981).

Beyond the key knowledge elements needed for navigating an organization, the blending of knowledge and skill are critical when seeking to assess the culture of the organization (e.g. traditions, values, rituals, flex-time, staff involvement in decision-making, teamwork) as well as the climate of the organization (e.g. work overload, continuous change in social policies, support in times of stress, rewards to counterbalance burnout). The knowledge associated with navigating an organization takes on increased significance in the midst of change (e.g. the exiting of an agency director or supervisor and an entering of new organizational leadership, contraction and expansion of agency funding and new social policies that call for new staff skills and training, and renewed calls for organizational reassessment and strategic planning) (Gibelman & Furman, 2008). The individual skills needed for coping with change parallel those used with clients (using a strengths-empowerment-advocacy perspective) can also be used with organizations in ways that promote and facilitate growth and change. A proactive, teamwork orientation is essential for engaging in organizational problem-solving, for designing small-scale changes that can grow to organization-wide implementation, and for the courage and candor to engage in the measurement of outcomes and the implementation of findings.

The practice wisdom associated with the successful navigation of human service organizations is captured by Gibelman and Furman (2008) in Figure 6. The themes relate to managing the scale of desired change, understanding and utilizing the chain of command, mobilizing others can lead to change, and the central role that personal and interpersonal relations play in the improvement of organizational life.

Organizational Focus

- Individual practitioners or groups of practitioners should determine which aspects of organizational work they wish to change; not everything can be on the agenda
- The appropriate chain of command should be followed in seeking an organizational response to an issue or problem
- Informal centers of power and influence can be mobilized to address some workplace issues, particularly those of an interpersonal nature
- The need to deal with difficult colleagues is a problem that emerges in all work environments
- Professional ethics include an obligation to work toward the improvement of the organization
- Realistic expectations about work in organizations are important determinants of the degree of personal satisfaction that may be derived

Personal/Interpersonal Focus

- Collegial relationships can be a positive or negative influence on staff attitudes toward the job and the organization
- The expertise of social workers in human relations and problem-solving can be applied to the resolution of workplace issues, using a broad conception of one's role rather than a minimalist perspective
- Mentoring can have an important influence on one's attitude and career development within the organization
- Career mobility within social work tends to be associated with movement from one organization to another
- The decision to stay or leave an organization is personal and depends on the level of satisfaction one derives from the current employment setting and one's overall career aspirations

Figure 6. Elements of improving organizational life*.
*Gibelman & Furman (2008, p. 225).

Shared core skills

When considering the skills shared by both micro and macro practitioners, several verbal and writing skills can be identified. In the area of verbal communications, the skills of active listening and engagement are as essential for worker–client relations as they are for staff–staff relations. The same is true for public presentation skills with a group of parents at a school or a group of staff at an inter-agency planning committee. The skills of reading and responding to an audience are often enhanced with the use of powerpoint presentation skills. Irrespective of one's position in an organization, the capacity to engage in perceptive observations about human behavior represents another communications skill.

In addition to interactional skills, the analytic skills that often appear in writing are also important for any form of practice. These clear and concise writing skills are often reflected in case records or meeting minutes, capacities for developing persuasive argumentation that often includes critical thinking skills, and a core set of problem-solving skills that reflect multi-level assessment (micro, mezzo, and macro perspectives).

While the differences between micro and macro practice are evident in organizational life, more attention is needed in explicating the commonalities across both domains of social work practice. Such *common* or shared skills include: a) relationship building (e.g. engagement, trust-building, collaboration), b) assessment (e.g. interaction between person and environment), c) promoting helping processes and engaging in change strategies (e.g. contracting and monitoring the change process), and d) effective use of self in fostering client empowerment use of empathy and cultural sensitivity. These *common* skills are of equal importance to the education of clinicians and community practitioners.

Many of these shared skills can be viewed as part of core social work competencies when they provide a foundation for more specialized skills needed by micro practitioners working with increasingly complex client issues or macro practitioners using their organizing, managing, or policy analysis skills. Each level of practice in a human service organization needs to acquire a comprehensive understanding of the skills and orientations of practitioners who have acquired different knowledge and skills. Similar to a case conference in a school that includes teachers, social workers, psychologists, nurses, reading specialists, and others it is helpful to know how each was educated in order to understand and engage the talents and experiences of others. All of these skills are needed in order to minimize the "blame game" that can emerge in some organizations where line staff complain about upper management and similar complaints can be found among managers when line staff do not appreciate the connections between case record documentation and agency financial accountability (Ezell, Chernesky, & Healy, 2004).

Micro-macro complementarity

In addition to shared core skills, micro practitioners clearly complement the work of macro practitioners and the same is true in reverse. Complementarity is an important aspect of the relationship between micro and macro practice. This section identifies some of the dimensions of this complementarity (Austin et al., 2016).

To begin, micro practice contributes in many ways to the success of macro practitioners. The contributions include the important role of self-awareness when it comes to the "effective use of self" in both micro and macro practice relationships. Similarly, the language of the helping and social change profession of social work provides an overall theme for interventions at all levels of practice. The articulation of problem-solving frameworks, both clinical and managerial, represent another area of complementarity. Another dimension of self-awareness is the role of self-reflective practice as an important ingredient for monitoring interventions at all levels of practice. And finally, since micro and macro practitioners engage in theory-informed practice, it is important to note the role of human behavior in the social environment. While it is well understood that human behavior is impacted by the social environment (especially social/environmental problems) and that human behavior can influence the social environment (empowerment), the interaction between these micro and macro dimensions of social science theory is less well understood. It is this bi-directional reciprocal impact between human behavior and the social environment that provides another dimension of micro-macro complementarity (Stone, Austin, Berzin, & Taylor, 2007).

When considering the complementary impact of macro practice on micro practice, we can see a shared commitment to theory-informed practice even though the micro form of practice tends to focus on the human behavior of client populations and the macro form of practice tends to focus on the social environment. There is also a shared commitment to leadership where micro practitioners advance to clinical leadership in the form of building upon practice experience to become a supervisor, trainer, coach, or senior manager. Leadership is an inherent part of macro practice when it comes to leading community organizing activities, serving as a program manager, or engaging in policy practice involved with advocacy, coalition-building, and/or lobbying. Given the interest among macro practitioners in evaluating services in order to improve decision-making and program development, similar interests can be found among micro practitioners when it comes to evidence-informed practice and identifying what works best for different client situations.

The focus of macro practitioners on the community provides another venue for identifying complementarity. For example, the search for the best way to prevent client problems involves the identification of prevention strategies and programs. This often calls for shifting the focus from individual clients to client populations in order to search "upstream" to locate critical opportunities to address social problems (e.g. gang violence, child abuse, elder abuse, slide into poverty, etc.). Prevention services often involve multiple agency participants, seed funding to test a new idea, investments in planning and evaluation, and commitment from all levels of staff.

An equally challenging arena relates to increasing the involvement of service users in agency decision-making. Efforts to amplifying the voices of service users in order to identify new ways to address the changing needs of clients can test the creativity and endurance of both micro and macro practitioners (Carnochan & Austin, 2015). Investing in this long-term process relates directly to identifying client empowerment approaches that helps communities address common needs and often calls for the redirection of existing staff and financial resources.

Conclusion

The opportunity to reflect and comment on one's life work is both a joy and a privilege as one approaches the 50-year milestone. While there are many challenges facing those of us invested in promoting macro social work practice, there is room for hope as the macro practice domain of the profession moves toward 20% of the graduates of university social work programs. As our knowledge base proliferates and the competition from other macro practice professions increases, it has become increasingly clear that curriculum consolidation and integration has become critical to opening up new "curricular shelf-space" for new knowledge and innovative practices.

This commentary began with the consolidation theme related to integrating the three domains of macro practice following decades of specialization and knowledge development. Students interested in systems change need an array of skills in order to address the contemporary challenges of service integration, amplify service user voices, promote innovation, measure service outcome, and build community in our urban and rural areas. In an effort to define macro practice, renewed emphasis was placed in this commentary on the managing aspects of community practice and the organizing aspects of management practice along with a continuing focus on policy practice that features the development, advocacy and implementation of social policies, often within the context of coalitions. This emphasis also features a renewed focus on social work macro practice in various education programs by reaffirming the preparation of students for professional practice within an ethics and social justice framework that is based on theory-informed practice, policy-informed practice, research evidence-informed practice, and diversity-informed practice.

As McBeath (2016) has noted, the principles that can guide the future developments of macro practice can be organized in terms of both internal and external dimensions. The external dimensions include developing external networks, strengthening agency-university practice partnerships, developing interdisciplinary initiatives for shared knowledge development, using technology to promote networks and to advocate, and the continuous scanning the environment for innovative policies, practices, and programs. Each of these external dimensions rely upon macro practice skills and processes. In addition, the dimensions internal to the social work professions include strengthening the linkages between micro, mezzo, and macro levels of practice, developing theory-informed macro practice, using equity-focused frameworks on human rights, and using evidence-informed macro practice.

The curricular implications of the three pathways identified in this commentary call for increased faculty dialog within the macro practice domain and throughout the social work curriculum. The Pathway 1 dialog agendas relate to developing new ways to integrate the traditional macro practice areas of community, management, and policy practice. The Pathway 2 agendas feature dialog between faculty with expertise in micro, mezzo, and macro practice when constructing advanced social work practice curricula. Finally, the Pathway 3 agendas call for faculty members who teach the foundation generalist practice courses to identify space for one or more modules that feature the interactions between micro and macro practice within at least two major contexts. These contexts include the interaction between human behavior and the social environment (e.g. client-neighborhood, service provider and service user, agency–environment interaction, and practitioner-environment) and the interaction between social policy and daily practice. If the space for macro practice in the foundation curriculum is limited, then the infusion of macro practice principles and practices needs to occur throughout the curriculum.

It is tempting to speculate on the future when macro social work practice continues to be viewed as an important component of social work practice. Conceptualizing future curricular structures calls for a transition from evidence-informed practice that focuses on the past (e.g. dates of references noted on most course outlines) to design-informed practice that focuses on the future (Cohen, 2011). Constructing scenarios is part of design thinking. Based on an understanding of macro practice as essential for all social work students, then the configuration of the current CSWE curriculum-focused competencies would need to be redesigned to feature the macro perspective before or in conjunction with the micro or mezzo perspectives. The following provide some examples of redesign thinking:

- *HBSE*: Reconfiguring the traditional life cycle construct for teaching about human behavior and the social environment by beginning with all aspects of the social environment that can impact human behavior (social problem perspective) as well as illustrations of how human behaviors can impact the social environment (client empowerment perspective). In essence, moving from the macro to the micro perspective.
- *Social Policy*: Reconfiguring the traditional historical construct used to help students understand policy-informed practice by beginning with the role of community-based advocacy and the evolution of coalitions in both policy development and policy implementation so that these macro practice issues provide a foundation for understanding the micro-practice-related policies (child safety in child welfare, harm to self or others in mental health, isolation in aging services, impacts of illness on self-sufficiency).
- *Generalist Social Work Practice*: Reconfiguring foundation practice courses in ways that feature the macro perspective in the beginning where examples of engagement, assessment, intervention, and evaluation feature organizational issues (changing the culture of the agency), community issues (amplifying the voices of service users) and policy advocacy issues (using the strengths perspective to empower self-help organizations).
- *Research*: Reconfigure the traditional description of the research enterprise that is often detached from other courses in order to introduce the parallel construction of the phases of intervention as they align with the phases of research (Austin & Isokuortti, 2016). The teaching of practice research provides a platform for integrating research and practice at the very beginning of the student's curriculum experience (Austin & Carnochan, 2019).
- *Intersectionality and Diversity*: Reconfiguring the traditional focus on client populations by exploring how these issues impact the staff in a human service agency, board members, elected

Specific Populations

- How do we identify baseline experiences and previously acquired skills of entering MSW students (both micro and macro) that provide a database for curriculum flexibility that contributes to building upon these experiences and skills?

  For decades, students have been frustrated by the assumptions underlying required social work courses that students are "blank slates" with very limited knowledge that needs to be acknowledged through standardized curricula. Can we hypothesize a difference between "blank slates" and "beginner's mindsets"?

- Given that most social work supervisors and managers have been promoted from the ranks of clinical/micro practice, what are the *core* macro practice skills needed by experienced practitioners and what types of innovative instructional approaches are needed to reach busy practitioners?

  Faculty accustomed to teaching introductory and advanced courses to students in their 20s will need a different approach (both content and processes) to teaching middle-managers in their 40s who bring substantial experience to the learning environment.

- How are the voices of service users amplified and incorporated into organizational and managerial decision-making?

  Rebalancing the power relationships between client populations and agency-based practitioners is an ongoing challenge for those engaged in macro practice. The voices of consumers are essential when moving from evidence-informed practice to design-informed practice.

- What are the processes and outcomes needed to engage macro practice faculty in curricular redesign related to integrating various forms of macro practice (community, management, and policy practice)? The same question applies to engaging micro and macro practice faculty in the search for cross-over competencies.

  Negotiating the sharing of cherished content buried in the course outlines of most faculty can be quite challenging, especially when others might be teaching content that formerly appeared in one's course. Again, design thinking is needed to reconfigure cherished content to make space for new content in an every changing practice environment.

Figure 7. Population and process research questions and rationales for macro practice education.

officials, and agency leaders. By focusing on the macro perspective before the micro practice issues, it is possible to help students see the institutionalized nature of oppression and discrimination before exploring how clients internalize various forms of trauma in the form of racism, sexism, homophobia, social class, agism, ablism and, more recently conceptualized, posttraumatic slave syndrome impacting African American males related, in part, to the increase in white supremacy and the excessive use of police force (St.Vil, St.Vil & Fairfax, 2019).

- *Interdisciplinary practice*: Given the increased interest in promoting interdisciplinary practice in many different fields of social work practice, how feasible would it be to require the completion of a course in another professional school outside of social work in order to graduate? While not all campuses would have professional schools of public health, public policy, law, education, journalism, criminology, business, medicine, nursing or urban planning, nearly all universities will have graduate programs in the social and behavioral sciences, as well as ethnic, racial and gender studies from which to draw.

Specific Processes

- How is the <u>changing nature of micro and macro practice</u> captured on a regular basis to inform curriculum updating processes?

  On the assumption that most social work faculty are some/many years removed from their prior practice experience (indeed, if there was such experience), it seems increasing urgent that annual conversations with relevant agency-practitioners be structured in the workload of campus-based faculty.

- How are new macro practice <u>skills incorporated into existing curriculum space</u> (e.g. data analytics and visualization, results-based management, performance enhancement tools, financial literacy associated with braided funding, etc.)?

  As in well-managed clothes closets, new clothing needs to replace some (not all) old clothing and this metaphor also applies to curricular space inside and outside existing courses. For example, the process of flipping the classroom experience from didactic to experiential has its own challenges when it comes to replacing the old with the new.

- How are <u>inter-disciplinary and intersectionality</u> content built into the learning environment of macro practice students?

  While each of these content areas are quite different from each other, they both call for the involvement of presenters with deep roots in either domain, not always reflected in the skill sets of campus-based faculty.

Figure 7. (Continued)

All of these examples seek to capture the use of design thinking when it comes to reconfiguring the entire social work curriculum in order to capture the element of macro practice that can inform micro and mezzo practice. There are multiple research questions that underlie these examples and several are noted in Figure 7 along with the respective rationales for each question.

The examples of design thinking also attempt to reinforce the macro dimensions of the "social" in social work when the vast majority of students declare their primary interests in working with individuals and families. As Reisch (2009, 2017) has noted over the past decade, the survival of macro practice is essential for the collective self-interest of the social work profession, especially in relationship to the profession's social justice mission that calls for using a "big picture" for addressing systemic inequalities and oppression.

Note 1: Some of the key community practice textbooks include the following: Ecklein and Lauffer (1972), Cox, Erlich, Rothman, and Tropman (1972), Perlman and Gurin (1972), Brager and Specht (1973), Rothman (1974), Rothman, Erlich, and Tropman (1974), Rothman, Erlich, and Teresa (1975), Grosser (1976), Cox, Erlich, Rothman, and Tropman (1977).

Note 2: Some of the key management practice textbooks include the following: Ehlers, Prothero, and Austin (1976), Trecker (1977), Slavin (1978), Tropman, Johnson, and Tropman (1979), Austin (1981), Weiner (1982), Hasenfeld (1983), Patti (1983), Skidmore (1983).

Disclosure statement

No potential conflict of interest was reported by the author.

References

Austin, M. J. (1981). *Supervisory management for the human services.* Englewood Cliffs, NJ: Prentice-Hall.

Austin, M. J. (1986). Community organization and social administration: Partnership or irrelevance? *Administration in Social Work, 10*(3), 27–39. doi:10.1300/J147v10n03_04

Austin, M. J. (1988). Managing up: Relationship building between middle management and top management. *Administration in Social Work, 12*(4), 29–46. doi:10.1300/J147v12n04_03

Austin, M. J. (2002). Managing out: The community practice dimensions of effective agency management. *Journal of Community Practice, 10*(4), 33–48. doi:10.1300/J125v10n04_03

Austin, M. J. (2018). Social work management practice (1917–2017): A history to inform the future. *Social Service Review, 92*(4), 548–616. doi:10.1086/701278

Austin, M. J., Anthony, E., Knee, T. R., & Mathias, J. (2016). Revisiting the relationship between micro and macro social work practice. *Families in Society, 97*(4), 270–277. doi:10.1606/1044-3894.2016.97.33

Austin, M. J., & Carnochan, S. (2019). *Practice research in the human services.* Berkeley: University of California, School of Social Welfare (publisher review pending).

Austin, M. J., Coombs, M., & Barr, B. (2005). Community-centered clinical practice: Searching for a continuum of micro and macro social work practice. *Journal of Community Practice, 13*(4), 9–30. doi:10.1300/J125v13n04_02

Austin, M. J., & Isokuortti, N. (2016). A framework for teaching practice-based research with a focus on service users. *Journal of Teaching in Social Work, Special Issue, 36*(1), 11–32. doi:10.1080/08841233.2016.1129931

Brager, G., & Specht, H. (1973). *Community organizing.* New York, NY: Columbia University Press.

Carnochan, S., & Austin, M. J. (2015). Redefining the bureaucratic encounter between service providers and service users: Evidence from the Norwegian HUSK Projects. *Journal of Evidence-based Social Work, 12*(1), 64–79.

Cohen, B. (2011). Design-based practice: A new perspective for social work. *Social Work, 56*(4), 337–346.

Council on Social Work Education. (2018). *Specialized practice curricular guide for macro social work practice.* Alexandria, VA: Author. Retrieved from https://www.cswe.org/CMSPages/GetFile.aspx?guid=553d03b4-c1f5-4f23-8241-a796edc6b922

Council on Social Work Education. (2019). *From social work education to social work practice: results of the survey of 2018 social work graduates.* Alexandria, VA: Author. https://www.cswe.org/CSWE/media/Workforce-Study/2018-Social-Work-Workforce-Report-Final.pdf?_zs=lGvTf1&_zl=O32h5

Cox, F., Erlich, J., Rothman, J., & Tropman, J. (Eds.). (1972). *Strategies of community organization – A book of readings.* Itasca, IL: Peacock Publishing.

Cox, F., Erlich, J., Rothman, J., & Tropman, J. (Eds.). (1977). *Tactics and techniques of community practice.* Itasca, IL: Peacock Publishing.

Donaldson, L. (2008). Developing a progressive advocacy program within a human services agency. *Administration in Social Work, 32*(2), 25–47. doi:10.1300/J147v32n02_03

Ecklein, J. L., & Lauffer, A. (1972). *Community organizers and social planners: Case and illustrative materials.* New York, NY: J. Wiley & Sons.

Ehlers, W., Prothero, J., & Austin, M. J. (1976). *Administration for the human service: An introductory programmed text.* New York, NY: Harper and Row.

Ezell, M. (2001). *Advocacy in the human services.* San Francisco, CA: Cengage Learning.

Ezell, M., Chernesky, R. H., & Healy, L. M. (2004). The learning climate for administration students. *Administration in Social Work, 28*(1), 57–76. doi:10.1300/J147v28n01_05

Fellin, P. (2001). *The community and the social worker* (3rd ed.). Itasca, IL: F. E. Peacock.

Fisher, R., & Corciullo, D. (2011). Rebuilding community organizing education in social work,". *Journal Of Community Practice, 19*(4), 355-368. doi:10.1080/10705422.2011.625537

Gibelman, M., & Furman, R. (2008). *Navigating human service organizations, 2nd ed.* Chicago, IL: Lyceum Books.

Grosser, C. (1976). *New directions in community organizing: From enabling to advocacy.* NY, USA: Praeger.

Gutierrez, L. M., & Gant, L. M. (2018). Community practice in social work: Reflections on its first century and directions for the future. *Social Service Review, 92*(4), 617–646. doi:10.1086/701640

Hardina. (2013). *Interpersonal social work skills for community practice.* New York, NY: Springer.

Hardina, D., Middleton, J., Montana, S., & Simpson, R. (2006). *An empowering approach to managing social service organizations.* New York, NY: Springer.

Hasenfeld, Y. (1983). *Human Service Organizations.* Englewood Cliffs, NJ: Prentice Hall.

Hernandez, V. R. (2008). Generalist and advanced generalist practice (pp. 260-268). In *Encyclopedia of social work.* Oxford, UK: Oxford University Press.

Jansson, B. (2014). *Becoming an effective policy advocate.* Belmont, CA: Brooks/Cole.

Kahn, A. (1969). *Theory and practice of social planning.* New York, NY: Russell Sage.

Kimberlin, S. E. (2010). Advocacy by nonprofits: Roles and practices of core advocacy organizations and direct service agencies. *Journal of Policy Practice, 9*(3–4), 164–182. doi:10.1080/15588742.2010.487249

Kramer, R. M., & Specht, H. (1969). *Readings in community organization practice.* Englewood Cliffs, NJ: Prentice-Hall.

Levi, D. (2018). *Group dynamics for teamwork* (5th ed.). Thousand Oaks, CA: Sage.

McBeath, B. (2016). Re-Envisioning macro social work practice. *Families in Society: the Journal of Contemporary Social Services, 97*(1), 5–14. doi:10.1606/1044-3894.2016.97.9

Menefee, D. (2009). What managers do and why they do it. In R. Patti (Ed.), *The handbook of human services management* (2nd ed., pp. 101–116). Thousand Oaks, CA: Sage.

Mott, A. (2008). Community Learning Project Report on University Education for Social Change. 2nd edition. Retrieved from www.communitylearningpartnership.org/strategy

Mulroy, E., & Austin, M. J. (2004). Towards a comprehensive framework for understanding the social environment: In search of theory for practice. *Journal of Human Behavior and the Social Environment, 10*(3), 25–59. doi:10.1300/J137v10n03_02

Netting, F. E., Kettner, P. M., McMurtry, S. L., & Thomas, L. (2017). *Social work macro practice* (6th ed.). Boston, MA: Pearson.

Network for Social Work Management. (2018). *Human services management competencies: A guide for nonprofit and for-profit agencies, foundations and institutions.* Los Angeles, CA: Author. Retrieved from https://socialworkmanager.org/wp-content/uploads/2018/12/HSMC-Guidebook-December-2018.pdf

Patti, R. (1983). *Social welfare administration: Managing social programs in a developmental context.* Englewood Cliffs, NJ: Prentice-Hall.

Perlman, R., & Gurin, A. (1972). *Community organization and social planning.* New York, NY: J. Wiley & Sons.

Reisch, M. (2009). General themes in the evolution of human services administration. In R. Patti (Ed.), *The handbook of human service management* (pp. 29–51). Thousand Oaks, CA: Sage.

Reisch, M. (2017). Why macro practice matters: Guest editorial. *Human Service Organizations: Management, Leadership & Governance, 41*(1), 6–9.

Reisch, M. (2018). *Macro practice social work: Working for change in a multi-cultural society.* San Diego, CA: Cognella Academic Publishing.

Rothman, J. (1974). *Planning and organizing for social change: Action principles from social science research.* New York, NY: Columbia University Press.

Rothman, J., Erlich, J., & Teresa, J. G. (1975). *Promoting innovation and change in organizations and communities: A planning manual.* NewYork, NY: J. Wiley & Sons.

Rothman, J., Erlich, J. L., & Tropman, J. F. (Eds.). (1974). *Strategies of community intervention.* Belmont, CA: Wadsworth/Thomson Learning.

Rothman, J., & Jones, W. C. (1971). *A new look at field instruction: Education for application of practice skills in community organization and social planning.* New York, NY: Association Press.

Schatz, H. A. (ed). (1970). *Social work administration: A resource book.* New York, NY: Council on Social Work Education.

Skidmore, R. A. (1983). *Social work administration: Dynamic management and human relationships.* Boston, MA, USA: Allyn & Bacon.

Slavin, S. (1978). *Social administration: The management of the social services.* New York, NY: Haworth Press.

Smale, G. C. (1995). Integrating community and individual practice: A new paradigm for practice. In Adams, P. and Nelson, K. (Eds.), *Reinventing human services,* Hawthorne, New York: Aldine de Gruyter.

St.Vil, St.Vil & Fairfax. (2019). Posttraumatic slave syndrome, the patriarchal nuclear family structure, and African American male–female relationships. *Social Work, 64*(2), 139–145. doi:10.1093/sw/swz002

Stone, D., Patton, B., & Heen, S. (1999). *Difficult conversations: How to discuss what matters most.* NY, USA: Penguin Group.

Stone, S., Austin, M. J., Berzin, A., & Taylor, S. (2007). Exploring the knowledge base of human behavior and the social environment using the concept of reciprocity. *Journal of Human Behavior and the Social Environment, 16*(3), 89–106. doi:10.1300/10911350802107769

Taylor, S., Austin, M. J., & Mulroy, E. (2004a). Social work textbooks on human behavior and the social environment: An analysis of the social environment component. *Journal of Human Behavior and the Social Environment, 10*(3), 85–109. doi:10.1300/J137v10n03_04

Taylor, S., Austin, M. J., & Mulroy, E. (2004b). Evaluating the social environment component of social work courses on human behavior and the social environment. *Journal of Human Behavior and the Social Environment, 10*(3), 61–84. doi:10.1300/J137v10n03_03

Toseland, R. W., & Rivas, R. F. (2017). *An introduction to group work practice* (8th ed.). New York, USA: Pearson.

Trecker, H. B. (1977). *Social work administration: Principles and practices* (2nd ed.). New York, NY: Association Press.

Tropman, J. E., Johnson, H., & Tropman, E. J. (1979). *Essentials of committee management.* Chicago, IL, USA: Nelson-Hall.

VeneKlasen, L., & Miller, V. (2007). *A new weave of power, people & politics: The action guide for advocacy and citizen participation.* Warwickshire, UK: Practical Action.

Weil, M. (Ed) (2005). *Handbook of community practice.* Thousand Oaks, CA: Sage Publications.

Weiner, M. (1982). *Human service management: Analysis and application.* Homewood, IL: Dorsey Press.

Whitaker, T., & Arrington, P. (2008). Social workers at work. In *NASW membership workforce study.* Washington, DC: National Association of Social Workers.

Implementation Science and Human Service Organizations Research: Opportunities and Challenges for Building on Complementary Strengths

Alicia C. Bunger ⓘ and Rebecca Lengnick-Hall

ABSTRACT

Implementation science (IS) and human service organizations (HSO) research both explore service quality and organizational impact in service of producing actionable evidence for leaders and managers. We believe there is potential to improve HSO quality and impact by working at the intersection of IS and HSO research. However, the strategic opportunities for integrating the unique strengths of these fields have not yet been fully explored, articulated, or leveraged. As HSOs encounter more pressure to implement evidence-based practices (EBPs), and IS continues to expand into new settings, now is the time for dialogue and collaboration among scholars in both fields. In this commentary, we share our vision for collaborative research that improves service quality and HSO impact. We discuss several strategic learning opportunities presented by this disciplinary intersection, identify specific recommendations for drawing on HSO and IS for study design, and consider challenges that face this research agenda.

Human service organizations (HSOs) play a vital role in improving the lives of individuals, families, groups, and communities. HSOs scholarship focuses on structures, technologies, processes, workforce dynamics, policies, environments, and strategies that shape the effectiveness and impact of these organizations. Yet, effectiveness and impact may be called into question when HSOs deliver services that are of poor or unknown quality. In response, we have seen a rise in policy and administrative tools that incentivize or reward HSOs for delivering evidence-based programs, practices, and models (EBPs) (e.g., Aarons, Hurlburt, & Horwitz, 2011; Collins-Camargo, McBeath, & Ensign, 2011; Powell et al., 2012). Today's HSO leaders and policymakers need to understand how to support and manage EBP implementation.

Implementation science (IS) emerged from similar quality concerns in healthcare. With substantial investment from major public healthcare agencies like the National Institutes of Health, IS has thrived since 2006. Although policy implementation in human services has been addressed in the public affairs literature (e.g., Pressman & Wildavsky, 1973), healthcare-focused IS aims to improve quality by focusing on EBP adoption, implementation, and sustainment (Eccles & Mittman, 2006; Roll, Moulton, & Sandfort, 2017). Specifically, IS (1) identifies quality gaps (assesses the degree to which services delivered in the real world are consistent with standards of care or EBPs); (2) explores implementation barriers and facilitators; (3) examines factors associated with implementation outcomes; and (4) tests implementation strategies (deliberate methods or interventions for integrating EBPs). IS generates new knowledge about the behavior of professionals, leaders, teams, organizations, and systems (e.g., Aarons et al., 2011). However, the applicability of these insights to leadership, management, and governance in diverse HSO settings remains unclear. While some settings (e.g., child welfare, juvenile justice, housing, and behavioral health) are increasingly represented in IS, many are not. A recent review by Roll et al. (2017) revealed that out of 1,507 implementation-related papers published across IS, public affairs, and related journals between 2004–2013, only 8% were set within social welfare settings (traditional human service domains), whereas 49% were set within healthcare and 18% in education.

Compared to healthcare organizations, HSOs must deliver highly complex services while mitigating acute capacity challenges (Despard, 2016; Proctor, 2014). Translating existing insights and generating new IS knowledge requires attention to the unique features of this context. First, many clients' human service needs extend beyond the scope or expertise of a single HSO, requiring coordination across multiple organizations that operate in siloed systems (e.g., behavioral health, child welfare, housing, domestic violence). This stands in contrast to healthcare organizations (e.g., hospitals, primary care clinics, skilled nursing facilities) that offer discrete treatments and address multiple health concerns under the same roof or system umbrella. Second, core human service technologies can be hard to define, describe, and measure since they are "inherently indeterminate, and ambiguous" (Sandfort, 2003, p. 606). This presents challenges when specifying intervention components, and delineating which ones are most important for improving client outcomes versus components that can be adapted.

Third, human services are delivered by a heterogeneous group of public, nonprofit, and for-profit organizations. Each actor within this organizational network has its own resource dependencies, structures, and capabilities (Chuang, Collins-Camargo, McBeath, Wells, & Bunger, 2014; Grønbjerg, 2001). HSOs often balance multiple services financed through a number of public and private funding sources each imposing their own (and sometimes competing) requirements. Fourth, human services are delivered in highly institutionalized and multi-level contexts. Practitioners are nested within teams, organizations, networks, regional systems, policy environments, and so on. Each contextual layer intersects and shapes the implementation of EBPs (Aarons et al., 2011; Greenhalgh, Robert, Macfarlane, Bate, & Kyriakidou, 2004; Moullin, Dickson, Stadnick, Rabin, & Aarons, 2019). As Aarons et al. (2011) note, this complexity makes EBP implementation and quality improvement in HSOs especially challenging compared to other contexts. Consequently, the lessons learned about EBP implementation in healthcare settings may not always be directly applicable to HSOs.

We believe there is potential to improve HSO quality and impact by working at the intersection of IS and HSO research. Both IS and HSO scholars share a mutual interest in helping leaders, managers, and practitioners create organizational environments that support the sustained use of effective services. However, the strategic opportunities for integrating the unique strengths of these fields have not yet been fully explored, articulated, or leveraged. As HSOs encounter more pressure to implement EBPs, and IS expands into new service settings, now is the time for dialog and collaboration among scholars in both fields. In this commentary, we first discuss several strategic opportunities for learning at this disciplinary intersection (Table 1). Second, we present six recommendations for drawing on the strengths of IS and HSO research in future studies that focus on EBP implementation in HSOs (Table 2). We conclude with a discussion of challenges and next steps for this HSO-IS research agenda.

Strategic opportunities for integrating IS and HSO research strengths

Expanding knowledge of the external organizational environment

Bridging IS and HSO scholarship will expand what we know about how the external organizational environment shapes EBP adoption, implementation, and sustainment. Both research streams share an interest in understanding and explaining ways in which systems and organizations influence service delivery. However, the external organizational environment – which is characterized as "outer setting" factors in popular IS frameworks (Damschroder et al., 2009) – has received limited empirical attention in IS. In IS, we know little about how or why the environment (e.g., institutional pressures, resource fluctuations, accrediting demands, competing interests, interorganizational relationships, and politics) influences organizations, teams, and practitioner behavior during implementation (Birken et al., 2017). Consequently, there is a need to expand insights about the specific ways the organizational environment can explain implementation outcomes.

HSO scholars have a strong understanding of the influence of external environments and pressures, which is needed to expand theory and knowledge in IS. For instance, recent research examined how HSOs respond to funding fluctuations, regulatory pressures, interorganizational relationships, and contracting arrangements (e.g., Collins-Camargo, Chuang, McBeath, & Mak, 2019; Lengnick-Hall, 2019; Park & Mosley, 2017). This work highlighted the complex and often nonlinear impact of environmental change and offered insights about how well-intended policy and professional pressure to demonstrate impact can have unintended consequences for organizations and communities (e.g., Mosley & Rathgeb Smith, 2018). HSOs and social workers experience tensions when these demands (e.g., to use an EBP, gather a specific quality metric) feel misaligned with their mission and practice (e.g., Bosk, 2018; Spitzmueller, 2018), leading some to actively resist. This critical lens is valuable for reframing how IS scholars understand organizational "resistance" to external implementation pressures and focuses our attention on aligning policy and institutional environments so that they support quality and impact across every level of the system.

HSO scholars' work reflects deep familiarity with a range of relevant theories (e.g., organizational structures, strategy, management, institutions, ecology), which are also necessary for advancing multi-level causal theories (i.e., theories that explain how factors at one level of the system impact those at another). Theory is essential in both IS and HSO research for organizing and synthesizing findings across diverse service settings. Multi-level causal theories are particularly important in IS for understanding and predicting how changes in the organizational environment lead to organizational, team, practitioner, and client outcomes (Lewis et al., 2018). HSO scholars are well positioned to help. For example, organizational scholars have considered how group or team-level climate and culture mediate the effect of organizational context on clinician behavior (Glisson & James, 2002; Zohar & Luria, 2005) or the reinforcing effect of interpersonal and interorganizational trust (Zaheer, McEvily, & Perrone, 1998). However, more work is needed in HSO scholarship as well, with continued calls to organizational scholars to build theories that bridge levels of the organizational ecosystem (Hitt, Beamish, Jackson, & Mathieu, 2007; Rousseau, 1985). Examining EBP implementation in HSO organizations offers opportunities to test multi-level causal theories and advance both HSO and IS research.

Developing relevant organizational and system-level interventions/tools

Bridging IS and HSO scholarship will support the development of effective organizational and system interventions and tools to support EBP implementation in human services. Although HSO scholars often observe and investigate managerial and administrative strategies, intervention development and testing have not been a central focus. IS, on the other hand, has a heavy interventional focus and aims to develop effective strategies for implementing EBPs. Many strategies target systems (e.g., changing policies, accreditation, funding) or organizations (e.g., create new teams, generate buy-in/support) (Powell et al., 2012, 2015; Proctor et al., 2009; Waltz et al., 2014). For instance, the Availability, Responsiveness, and Continuity (ARC) intervention was designed to improve organizational culture and climate within children's service organizations (Glisson, Dukes, & Green, 2006), and serves as an effective strategy for implementing EBPs (Glisson et al., 2010). Other organizational interventions – such as Leadership and Organizational Change for Implementation (LOCI), a leadership consultation intervention – are designed to improve leadership behaviors, climate, and implementation outcomes (Aarons, Ehrhart, Moullin, Torres, & Green, 2017).

The expansion of EBP implementation into human service settings will require additional interventions and pragmatic tools tailored for HSOs. HSO scholars are well-positioned to advance these types of strategies given their interests in management and administration. For instance, Tollarová and Furmaníková (2017) highlight personnel management strategies used to support organizational change including staff hiring, development, scheduling, and workplace design. Considering the importance of policy, regulations, and public funding for human services, traditional public management strategies (e.g., mandates, financial incentives or penalties, network coordination, professional requirements) are also strategies that can be used to promote implementation. Translating what we know about these approaches (from the HSO literature) to IS can expand the implementation strategies and tools that target organizations and systems, particularly among HSOs.

Improving research rigor

HSO and IS have complementary methodological strengths that can improve research rigor. First, strong IS research designs for testing interventions help fill the acknowledged need for more rigorous organizational research designs (Aguinis, Pierce, Bosco, & Muslin, 2008). IS has brought attention to a range of quasiexperimental research designs. Clustered controlled trials, stepped wedge designs, sequential multiple assignment randomized trials (SMART) and other approaches for understanding organizational and system changes grow more common each year (Brown et al., 2017; Mazzucca et al., 2018). These quasiexperimental approaches from IS could be useful for examining the effects of policy, institutional, or organizational changes (beyond implementation) in HSO settings. They promote internal validity (longitudinal measures, comparison groups) while embracing many of the real-world exigencies of conducting organizational research (nesting within teams or organizations, staggering recruitment over time, or the need to ensure the entire organizational population benefits from the intervention).

Second, HSO scholars have methodological strengths that are directly useful for IS studies in HSO settings. For example, HSO scholarship has considered sampling approaches within complex

Table 1. Challenges and complementary strengths of human service organization and implementation of science research.

	Challenges	Strengths
Expanding Knowledge and Theory	IS: • External organizational environment has received limited empirical attention. • Need for multi-level causal theories to elaborate multi-level mechanisms of change.	HSOs: • Understanding the influence of external environments and pressures. • Deep familiarity with a range of organizational theories.
	HSOs: • Bridging theoretical traditions and levels.	IS: • Opportunity and platform for studying the multilevel system and organizational changes.
Developing Relevant Organizational Interventions & Tools	IS: • Expanding strategies that target systems, organizations, and management.	HSOs: • Examining the role of a variety of management and public management approaches.
	HSOs: • Translating research findings into HSO-relevant interventions and tools and testing effectiveness.	IS: • Heavy focus on strategy development and testing.
Improving Research Rigor	IS: • Increasing interest in rigorous approaches to capturing organizational-level constructs.	HSOs: • Specialized expertise in sampling, measures, data aggregation, and ethical issues in organizational research.
	HSOs: • Rigorous organizational research designs.	IS: • Refined set of quasiexperimental designs.

settings, measures of organizational constructs, and data aggregation issues. IS can also benefit from HSO scholars' expertise in navigating unique ethical issues and participant risks in organizational research. Employee participation is common in both IS and HSO research, and proper privacy/confidentiality safeguards are necessary to protect employees from retaliation and from having their participation status or responses used to evaluate their performance. Finally, HSO scholars offer extensive expertise in qualitative methods for examining organizational and system conditions. For example, Spitzmueller's (2018) thorough ethnography elucidated the consequences of tensions between the managerial logic (which emphasize standardization and performance measurement) and front-line logic (which prioritizes self-determination and collaboration) as an organization experienced transformational change. The range of qualitative methods commonly used in HSO research (e.g., ethnography, phenomenological studies, in-depth multiple case studies, document reviews, elicitation approaches) is useful for IS and consistent with recent calls for the field to move beyond interviews and focus groups (QUALRIS, 2019).

Recommendations for designing studies that integrate HSO and IS scholarship

To illustrate our vision for research that draws on both fields to improve HSO quality and impact, we explore six recommendations (Table 2).

1. *HSO-IS research studies should examine implementation within the context of regional systems. The regional system is the unit of analysis.* To date, many implementation studies focus on discrete organizations, and clinicians within them, without accounting sufficiently for how the larger external environment and relationships among organizations influence implementation. HSO-IS studies might focus on regional systems as a whole. For example, examining the implementation of multiple EBPs throughout Philadelphia's mental health system highlighted the complex interactions among organizational and system stakeholders, the policy environment, and environmental pressures (e.g., Beidas et al., 2013, 2015; Powell et al., 2016). Building upon Aarons' and colleagues' longstanding program of SafeCare implementation research, Lengnick-Hall (2019) examined how organizations adapted in response to a child welfare intervention relative to other peer organizations in the same service system. Moving the focus to the outer levels of the service delivery ecosystem opens the door for more direct investigation of how organizational decisions to adopt and implement EBPs are influenced by relationships with peer organizations, public agencies, client advocacy groups, private funders (e.g., the United Way), and accrediting bodies.

2. *HSO-IS studies should advance and test data-driven, multi-level implementation decision-making processes.* Strategies that are effective in one organization may not be effective in another; effective implementation depends on the selection of strategies that address the unique contextual strengths and challenges. Instead of focusing on the effectiveness of a specific implementation strategy (or combinations thereof), HSO-IS studies might test approaches that help managers and leaders select implementation strategies that fit their organization or system (Powell et al., 2019). This type of approach might incorporate an assessment of system strengths and opportunities, followed by data-informed selection of implementation strategies that target identified needs. For instance, Powell, Aarons, Amaya-Jackson, Haley, and Weiner (2018) are piloting the Collaborative Organizational Approach to Selecting and Tailoring Implementation Strategies (COAST-IS), a multi-phase process that engages stakeholder wisdom, theory, and evidence. Examining the feasibility and effectiveness of decision-making processes or models may be especially relevant to human service leaders and administrators managing change in such complex environments.

3. *HSO-IS studies should use mixed-methods and rigorous quasiexperimental designs.* Building evidence about the multi-level context and interventions that promote EBP implementation in HSO settings will likely require quasiexperimental studies, with the regional service delivery system as the focal

unit. Contemporary IS studies and prior behavioral health system demonstration evaluations point to relevant designs for examining organizational and system changes that draw on both qualitative and quantitative data to triangulate information across stakeholders. For instance, matched-pair clustered trial could be used to evaluate the effects of system interventions, where city or regional systems are paired based on similar contextual features, and randomized to study conditions (e.g., Randolph et al., 2002). When interventions cannot be withheld from a system, stepped wedge trials might be useful (where implementation is rolled out in stages across states or regions) (e.g., Chamberlain et al., 2008). Stepped wedge or other types of adaptive designs allow study stakeholders to refine their implementation approach and create comparison conditions within naturally occurring policy or practice initiatives. These designs are especially useful for leveraging naturally occurring implementation efforts such as new policies requiring EBP implementation funding fluctuations, or other shocks to the system that influence resources, interests, and political will. At the same time, hybrid studies – those that examine the effectiveness of the implementation approach *and* the EBP – could be especially useful in human services, where many interventions, programs, and models have not yet been subjected to rigorous effectiveness tests (Curran, Bauer, Mittman, Pyne, & Stetler, 2012). If these designs are not feasible because of sample demands, multiple case studies with rich qualitative and quantitative data (e.g., Aarons, Fettes, Sommerfeld, & Palinkas, 2012; Morrissey et al., 1994; Provan & Milward, 1995) can address questions related to implementation outcomes with smaller numbers of systems.

4. *HSO-IS studies should emphasize relationships with community partners.* Research that blends HSO and IS strengths likely involves advanced and long-term commitments to partnering with community stakeholders. HSO scholars are often steeped in a strong tradition of applied and community-engaged scholarship that is applicable to understanding implementation (Adams, 2018; Palinkas, He, Choy-Brown, & Hertel, 2017). Engaging community partners can help orient the team to practice-relevant research questions, identify innovations in the field, collaboratively address potential participant burden, develop creative ways to incentivize and sustain participant buy-in (and manage turnover), and cue the team to the dynamics, conflicts, information asymmetry, and power differentials among participants (Chambers & Azrin, 2013; Palinkas et al., 2017; Palinkas, Short, & Wong, 2015). Such close engagement is also useful for understanding service inequities, intervention adaptations within the broader service ecosystem, and client engagement. Finally, crafting evidence-informed policy and funding recommendations also necessitates ongoing communication with knowledgeable stakeholders.

5. *HSO-IS studies should examine implementation costs.* HSOs operate under significant financial constraints that limit quality improvements like EBP implementation, especially in small HSOs (Bunger, Despard, Lee, & Cao, 2019; Despard, 2016). High costs associated with EBPs and their implementation are a critical consideration for HSO leaders; however, these costs have received little empirical attention in IS. HSO-IS studies will likely document direct and indirect implementation costs, develop low-cost tools, conduct economic evaluations of implementation strategies, and consider long-term return-on-investment for organizations and systems. Understanding the economic impacts and value of implementation is critical for informing HSO leaders' and policy-makers' investment decisions (Eisman, Kilbourne, Dopp, Saldana, & Eisenberg, 2019).

6. *HSO-IS studies should be translated for and disseminated to diverse audiences.* HSO-IS studies are intended to inform research and practice (broadly defined); thus, our results must be translated and disseminated to multiple audiences. However, policymakers, organizational leaders, frontline staff, and client advocacy groups have different information needs than traditional academic audiences. This requires us to work with our stakeholders to disseminate findings in accessible and usable formats. Examples include practical guides, toolkits, decision supports, white papers, and research briefs in everyday language. We might also consider making data-informed recommendations when appropriate (e.g., policy recommendations at the local, state, and federal levels).

Table 2. Design recommendations for scholars working at the intersection of human service organization and implementation science research.

	Design Recommendations
Expanding Knowledge and Theory	• Consider the human service system as focal unit (rather than organizations or clinicians only). • Thorough assessment of context. • Longitudinal studies (to examine implementation amidst environmental fluctuations and shocks).
Developing Relevant Organizational Interventions & Tools	• Test the feasibility and effectiveness of data-driven, multi-level decision-making processes (rather than discrete implementation strategies). • Community-engaged studies. • Consider cost.
Improving Research Rigor	• Rigorous quasiexperimental, multimethod, and hybrid studies.

Challenges

We recognize that an HSO-IS research agenda will require ambitious large-scale studies, significant and sustained resources, and multi-disciplinary teams with strong community partnerships. We anticipate three general challenges for an HSO-IS research agenda. First, organizational- and system-level studies often suffer from analysis challenges. Even large-scale studies of organizations and systems may have insufficient sample sizes for rigorous statistical analysis, and while case studies generate important insights, causal inference is limited. To push the science forward, scholars might need to pursue alternative approaches that optimize small or medium-sized samples (such as qualitative comparative analysis) (Rihoux & Ragin, 2009), or system science approaches that simulate policy, funding, or other environmental scenarios that cannot be experimentally manipulated (Burke et al., 2015). This will require tailored training opportunities for students and scholars, as well as shifting social norms in the academic community about what constitutes rigorous analysis.

Second, scholars may need to tailor the selection, operationalization, and measurement of relevant implementation outcomes in HSOs. For instance, fidelity is a common implementation outcome that reflects the degree to which an intervention has been implemented as intended, and requires a clear delineation of key intervention components (Proctor et al., 2011). However, EBPs implemented in HSO settings are often complex, with multiple interdependent components that may have been adapted to fit the target population and the organizational setting. This makes conceptualization of the core components and their measurement very challenging. Scholars might consider breaking down an intervention into its core functions (intervention purpose) and forms (specific strategies tailored to the context), in collaboration with their community partners (Perez Jolles, Lengnick-Hall, & Mittman, 2019). This approach could help identify which intervention elements are most critical for impact (and thus, need to be measured to assess fidelity) and which elements can be adapted. Doing so may require scholars to revisit the conceptual underpinnings of interventions with developers.

Third, funding and support for this work are limited and highly competitive. Carrying out organizational- and system-level studies require substantial and sustained financial resources. Current IS funding and dissemination outlets offer the opportunity for HSO and IS scholars to advance implementation knowledge and practice in HSO settings. For instance, the National Institutes of Health has a dedicated IS funding stream (e.g., PAR-19-274, 275, 276), and the U.S. Children's Bureau also supported implementation evaluations in their demonstration projects (e.g., U.S. Department of Health and Human Services [USDHHS], 2012). These opportunities offer financial resources for assembling interdisciplinary teams and recruiting robust samples of organizations or systems for developing/testing theories and interventions. Expanding IS into a greater diversity of HSO settings will require comparable investment from other funders that support research and programming across different human service areas. Setting aside funding for implementation capacity building and evaluation might help move this work forward. However, we acknowledge that research funding often does not cover the deep and prolonged inter-disciplinary and community collaboration needed to yield a successful proposal, new data, or a published manuscript. Thus, HSO-IS scholars will also need substantial institutional support to build and nurture these relationships over time, and in between grants, while balancing pressures for traditional research productivity (Gopalan, Bunger, & Powell, 2019).

Concluding thoughts and next steps

While we recognize the ambitious and challenging nature of this work, advancing HSO-IS research has the potential to improve HSO quality and impact. We conclude with next steps for scholars interested in building bridges across disciplines. First, browse a journal outside of your dominant orientation (e.g., HSO scholars might read *Implementation Science*, IS scholars might read *Human Service Organizations: Management, Leadership, and Governance*). Second, familiarize yourself with an HSO or IS theory/framework that is new to you. Consider how it aligns with your research interests and could inform hypotheses, study design, or interventions. Third, explore how an HSO or IS audience shapes the focus, framing, and presentation of HSO-IS studies. Check the NIH RePORT (https://projectreporter.nih.gov/reporter.cfm) to identify new HSO-IS studies that have been funded. While you are online, scan abstracts from conferences on HSOs (e.g., Public Management Research Association, Network for Social Work Managers) or IS (e.g., Annual Conference on the Science of Dissemination and Implementation in Health, Society for Implementation Research and Collaboration). Finally, reach out to a new HSO or IS colleague and begin a dialogue around your shared research interests and goals. Within universities, HSO scholars may be dispersed across social work, public affairs, or business schools, while IS scholars may be concentrated in medical centers or schools of public health. Discussion topics may include current projects, pressing research questions in the field, preferred publication outlets, funding opportunities, organizing theories and frame-works, and stakeholder engagement. We look forward to the continued discussion and discovery with our academic and management colleagues as we realize these important synergies across fields.

Disclosure statement

No potential conflict of interest was reported by the authors.

ORCID

Alicia C. Bunger (iD) http://orcid.org/0000-0002-6407-5111

References

Aarons, G. A., Ehrhart, M. G., Moullin, J. C., Torres, E. M., & Green, A. E. (2017). Testing the leadership and organizational change for implementation (LOCI) intervention in substance abuse treatment: A cluster randomized trial study protocol. *Implementation Science*, 12(1), 29. doi:10.1186/s13012-017-0562-3

Aarons, G. A., Fettes, D. L., Sommerfeld, D. H., & Palinkas, L. A. (2012). Mixed methods for implementation research: Application to evidence-based practice implementation and staff turnover in community-based organizations providing child welfare services. *Child Maltreatment*, 17(1), 67–79. doi:10.1177/1077559511426908

Aarons, G. A., Hurlburt, M., & Horwitz, S. M. (2011). Advancing a conceptual model of evidence-based practice implementation in public service sectors. *Administration and Policy in Mental Health*, 38(1), 4–23. doi:10.1007/s10488-010-0327-7

Adams, D. R. (2018). Social work's role in collaborative community-academic partnerships. *Social Work*, 1–9. doi:10.1016/0038-1098(79)91043-3

Aguinis, H., Pierce, C. A., Bosco, F. A., & Muslin, I. S. (2008). First decade of organizational research methods. *Organizational Research Methods*, 12. doi:10.1177/1094428108322641

Beidas, R. S., Aarons, G., Barg, F., Evans, A., Hadley, T., Hoagwood, K., … Mandell, D. S. (2013). Policy to implementation: Evidence-based practice in community mental health–Study protocol. *Implementation Science, 8* (1), 38. doi:10.1186/1748-5908-8-38

Beidas, R. S., Marcus, S., Aarons, G. A., Hoagwood, K. E., Schoenwald, S., Evans, A. C., … Adams, D. R. (2015). Individual and organizational factors related to community clinicians' use of therapy techniques in a large public mental health system. *JAMA Pediatrics, 169*(4), 374. doi:10.1001/jamapediatrics.2014.3736

Birken, S. A., Bunger, A. C., Powell, B. J., Turner, K., Clary, A. S., Klaman, S. L., … Weiner, B. J. (2017). Organizational theory for dissemination and implementation research. *Implementation Science, 12*(1). doi:10.1186/s13012-017-0592-x

Bosk, E. A. (2018). What counts? quantification, worker judgment, and divergence in child welfare decision making. *Human Service Organizations: Management, Leadership & Governance, 42*(2), 205–224.

Brown, C. H., Curran, G., Palinkas, L. A., Aarons, G. A., Wells, K. B., Jones, L., … Cruden, G. (2017). An overview of research and evaluation designs for dissemination and implementation. *Annual Review of Public Health, 38*, 1–22. doi:10.1146/annurev-publhealth-031816-044215

Bunger, A. C., Despard, M., Lee, M., & Cao, Y. (2019). The cost of quality: Organizational financial health and program quality. *Journal of Evidence-Informed Social Work, 16*(1), 18–35. doi:10.1080/23761407.2018.1536575

Burke, J. G., Lich, K. H., Neal, J. W., Meissner, H. I., Yonas, M., & Mabry, P. L. (2015). Enhancing dissemination and implementation research using systems science methods. *International Journal of Behavioral Medicine, 22*(3), 283–291. doi:10.1007/s12529-014-9417-3

Chamberlain, P., Brown, C. H., Saldana, L., Reid, J., Wang, W., Marsenich, L., … Bouwman, G. (2008). Engaging and recruiting counties in an experiment on implementing evidence-based practice in California. *Administration and Policy in Mental Health, 35*(4), 250–260. doi:10.1007/s10488-008-0167-x

Chambers, D. A., & Azrin, S. T. (2013). Research and services partnerships: Partnership: A fundamental component of dissemination and implementation research. *Psychiatric Services, 64*(6), 509–511. doi:10.1176/appi.ps.201300032

Chuang, E., Collins-Camargo, C., McBeath, B., Wells, R., & Bunger, A. (2014). An empirical typology of private child and family serving agencies. *Children and Youth Services Review, 38*, 101–112. doi:10.1016/j.childyouth.2014.01.016

Collins-Camargo, C., Chuang, E., McBeath, B., & Mak, S. (2019). Staying afloat amidst the tempest: External pressures facing private child and family serving agencies and managerial strategies employed to address them. *Human Service Organizations: Management, Leadership & Governance, 43*(2), 125–145.

Collins-Camargo, C., McBeath, B., & Ensign, K. (2011). Privatization and performance-based contracting in child welfare: Recent trends and implications for social service administrators. *Administration in Social Work, 35*(5), 494–516. doi:10.1080/03643107.2011.614531

Curran, G. M., Bauer, M., Mittman, B., Pyne, J. M., & Stetler, C. (2012). Effectiveness-implementation hybrid designs: Combining elements of clinical effectiveness and implementation research to enhance public health impact. *Medical Care, 50*(3), 217–226. doi:10.1097/MLR.0b013e3182408812

Damschroder, L. J., Aron, D. C., Keith, R. E., Kirsh, S. R., Alexander, J. A., & Lowery, J. C. (2009). Fostering implementation of health services research findings into practice: A consolidated framework for advancing implementation science. *Implementation Science, 4*(50). doi:10.1186/1748-5908-4-50

Despard, M. R. (2016). Challenges in implementing evidence-based practices and programs in nonprofit human service organizations. *Journal of Evidence-informed Social Work, 13*(6), 505–522. doi:10.1080/23761407.2015.1086719

Eccles, M. P., & Mittman, B. S. (2006). Welcome to implementation science. *Implementation Science, 1*(1), 1. doi:10.1186/1748-5908-1-1

Eisman, A. B., Kilbourne, A. M., Dopp, A. R., Saldana, L., & Eisenberg, D. (2019). Economic evaluation in implementation science: Making the business case for implementation strategies. *Psychiatry Research.* doi:10.1016/j.psychres.2019.06.008

Glisson, C., Dukes, D., & Green, P. (2006). The effects of the ARC organizational intervention on caseworker turnover, climate, and culture in children's service systems. *Child Abuse & Neglect, 30*, 855–880. doi:10.1016/j.chiabu.2005.12.010

Glisson, C., & James, L. R. (2002). The cross-level effects of culture and climate in human service teams. *Journal of Organizational Behavior, 23*(6), 767–794. doi:10.1002/job.162

Glisson, C., Schoenwald, S. K., Hemmelgarn, A., Green, P., Dukes, D., Armstrong, K. S., & Chapman, J. E. (2010). Randomized trial of MST and ARC in a two-level evidence-based treatment implementation strategy. *Journal of Consulting and Clinical Psychology, 78*(4), 537–550. doi:10.1037/a0019160

Gopalan, G., Bunger, A. C., & Powell, B. J. (2019). Skills for developing and maintaining community-partnerships for dissemination and implementation research in children's behavioral health: Implications for research infrastructure and training of early career investigators. *Administration and Policy in Mental Health and Mental Health Services Research.* doi:10.1007/s10488-019-00930-5

Greenhalgh, T., Robert, G., Macfarlane, F., Bate, P., & Kyriakidou, O. (2004). Diffusion of innovations in service organizations: Systematic review and recommendations. *The Milbank Quarterly, 82*(4), 581–629. doi:10.1111/j.0887-378X.2004.00325.x

Grønbjerg, K. A. (2001). Grønbjerg U.S. nonprofit human service sector the U.S. nonprofit human service sector: A creeping revolution. *Nonprofit and Voluntary Sector Quarterly, 30*(2), 276–297. doi:10.1177/0899764001302006

Hitt, M. A., Beamish, P. W., Jackson, S. E., & Mathieu, J. E. (2007). Building theoretical and empirical bridges across levels: Multilevel research in management. *Academy of Management Journal, 50*(6), 1385–1399. doi:10.5465/amj.2007.28166219

Lengnick-Hall, R. (2019). *How organizations adapt during EBP implementation.* (Doctoral dissertation), University of Southern California, Los Angeles.

Lewis, C. C., Klasnja, P., Powell, B. J., Lyon, A. R., Tuzzio, L., Jones, S., … Weiner, B. (2018). From classification to causality: Advancing understanding of mechanisms of change in implementation science. *Frontiers in Public Health, 6*, 136. doi:10.3389/fpubh.2018.00136

Mazzucca, S., Tabak, R. G., Pilar, M., Ramsey, A. T., Baumann, A. A., Kryzer, E., … Brownson, R. C. (2018). Variation in research designs used to test the effectiveness of dissemination and implementation strategies: A review. *Frontiers in Public Health, 6*(February), 1–10. doi:10.3389/fpubh.2018.00032

Morrissey, J., Calloway, M. O., Bartko, W. T., Ridgely, M. S., Goldman, H. H., & Paulson, R. I. (1994). Local mental health authorities and service system change: Evidence from the Robert Wood Johnson foundation program on chronic mental illness. *The Millbank Quarterly, 72*(1), 49–80. doi:10.2307/3350338

Mosley, J. E., & Rathgeb Smith, S. (2018). Human service agencies and the question of impact: Lessons for theory, policy, and practice. *Human Service Organizations: Management, Leadership & Governance, 42*(2), 113–122.

Moullin, J.C., Dickson, K.S., Stadnick, N., Rabin, B, Aarons, G.A. (2019). Systematic review of the exploration, preparation, implementation, sustainment (EPIS) framework. *Implementation Science, 14*(1). https://doi.org/10.1186/s13012-018-0842-6.

Palinkas, L. A., He, A. S., Choy-Brown, M., & Hertel, A. L. (2017). Operationalizing social work science through research–practice partnerships. *Research on Social Work Practice, 27*(2), 181–188. doi:10.1177/1049731516666329

Palinkas, L. A., Short, C., & Wong, M. (2015). *Research-practice-policy partnerships for implementation of evidence-based practices in child welfare and child mental health* (Report prepared for the William T. Grant Foundation). Retrieved from http://wtgrantfoundation.org/resource/research-practice-policy-partnerships-for-implementation-of-evidence-based-practices-in-child-welfare-and-child-mental-health

Park, S. E., & Mosley, J. (2017). Nonprofit growth and decline during economic uncertainty. *Human Service Organizations: Management, Leadership & Governance, 41*(5), 515–531.

Perez Jolles, M., Lengnick-Hall, R., & Mittman, B. S. (2019). Core functions and forms of complex health interventions: A patient-centered medical home illustration. *Journal of General Internal Medicine*, 1–7. doi:10.1007/s11606-018-4818-7

Powell, B. J., Aarons, G. A., Amaya-Jackson, L., Haley, A., & Weiner, B. J. (2018). The collaborative approach to selecting and tailoring implementation strategies (COAST-IS). *Implementation Science, 13*(Suppl 3), A79, 39–40. doi:10.1186/s13012-018-0779-9

Powell, B. J., Beidas, R. S., Rubin, R. M., Stewart, R. E., Wolk, C. B., Matlin, S. L., … Mandell, D. S. (2016). Applying the policy ecology framework to Philadelphia's behavioral health transformation efforts. *Administration and Policy in Mental Health and Mental Health Services Research*, 1–18. doi:10.1007/s10488-016-0733-6

Powell, B. J., Fernandez, M. E., Williams, N. J., Aarons, G. A., Beidas, R. S., Lewis, C. C., … Weiner, B. J. (2019). Enhancing the impact of implementation strategies in healthcare: A research agenda. *Frontiers in Public Health, 7*, 3. doi:10.3389/fpubh.2019.00003

Powell, B. J., McMillen, J. C., Proctor, E. K., Carpenter, C. R., Griffey, R. T., Bunger, A. C., … York, J. L. (2012). A compilation of strategies for implementing clinical innovations in health and mental health. *Medical Care Research and Review : MCRR, 69*(2), 123–157. doi:10.1177/1077558711430690

Powell, B. J., Waltz, T. J., Chinman, M. J., Damschroder, L. J., Smith, J. L., Matthieu, M. M., … Kirchner, J. E. (2015). A refined compilation of implementation strategies: Results from the Expert Recommendations for Implementing Change (ERIC) project. *Implementation Science : IS, 10*(1), 21. doi:10.1186/s13012-015-0209-1

Pressman, J. L., & Wildavsky, A. (1973). *Implementation how great expectations in Washington are dashed in Oakland; or, why it's amazing that federal programs work at all, this being a saga of the economic development administration as told by two sympathetic observers who seek to build morals on.* Berkeley, CA, USA: University of California Press.

Proctor, E. (2014). Dissemination and Implementation Research. *Encyclopedia of Social Work.* doi:10.1093/acrefore/9780199975839.013.900

Proctor, E., Silmere, H., Raghavan, R., Hovmand, P., Aarons, G. A., Bunger, A., … Hensley, M. (2011). Outcomes for implementation research: Conceptual distinctions, measurement challenges, and research agenda. *Administration and Policy in Mental Health, 38*(2), 65–76. doi:10.1007/s10488-010-0319-7

Proctor, E. K., Landsverk, J., Aarons, G., Chambers, D., Glisson, C., & Mittman, B. (2009). Implementation research in mental health services: An emerging science with conceptual, methodological, and training challenges. *Administration and Policy in Mental Health, 36*(1), 24–34. doi:10.1007/s10488-008-0197-4

Provan, K. G., & Milward, H. B. (1995). A preliminary theory of interorganizational network effectiveness: A comparative study of four community mental health systems. *Administrative Science Quarterly, 40*(1), 1–33. doi:10.2307/2393698

QUALRIS. (2019). Qualitative Research in Implementation Science. Division of Cancer Control and Population Sciences, National Cancer Institute. https://cancercontrol.cancer.gov/IS/docs/NCI-DCCPS-ImplementationScience-WhitePaper.pdf.

Randolph, F., Blasinsky, M., Morrissey, J., Rosenheck, R. A., Cocozza, J., & Goldman, H. H. (2002). Overview of the ACCESS program. *Psychiatric Services*, *53*(8), 945–948. doi:10.1176/appi.ps.53.2.133

Rihoux, B., & Ragin, C. (2009). *Configurational comparative methods: Qualitative comparative analysis (QCA) and related techniques*. Thousand Oaks, CA: Sage Publications.

Roll, S., Moulton, S., & Sandfort, J. (2017). A comparative analysis of two streams of implementation research. *Journal of Public and Nonprofit Affairs*, *3*(1), 3. doi:10.20899/jpna.3.1.3-22

Rousseau, D. M. (1985). Issues of level in organizational research: Multi-level and cross-level perspectives. *Research in Organizational Behavior1*, *7*, 1–37.

Sandfort, J. R. (2003). Exploring the structuration of technology within human service organizations. *Administration & Society*, *34*(6), 605–631. doi:10.1177/0095399702239167

Spitzmueller, M. C. (2018). Remaking "community" mental health: Contested institutional logics and organizational change. *Human Service Organizations: Management, Leadership & Governance*, *42*(2), 123–145.

Tollarová, B., & Furmaníková, L. (2017). Personnel strategies in the deinstitutionalization process: How do the managers work with employees? *Human Service Organizations: Management, Leadership & Governance*, *41*(5), 532–559.

U.S. Department of Health and Human Services. (2012). *Initiative to improve access to needs-driven, evidence-based /evidence-informed mental and behavioral health services in child welfare*.

Waltz, T. J., Powell, B. J., Chinman, M. J., Smith, J. L., Matthieu, M. M., Proctor, E. K., … Kirchner, J. E. (2014). Expert recommendations for implementing change (ERIC): Protocol for a mixed methods study. *Implementation Science*, *9* (39), 1. doi:10.1186/1748-5908-1-1

Zaheer, A., McEvily, B., & Perrone, V. (1998). Does trust matter? Exploring the effects of interorganizational and interpersonal trust on performance. *Organization Science*, *9*(2), 141–159. doi:10.1287/orsc.9.2.141

Zohar, D., & Luria, G. (2005). A multilevel model of safety climate: Cross-level relationships between organization and group-level climates. *Journal of Applied Psychology*, *90*(4), 616–628. doi:10.1037/0021-9010.90.4.616

We Could Be Unicorns: Human Services Leaders Moving from Managing Programs to Managing Information Ecosystems

Lauri Goldkind ⓘ and John G. McNutt ⓘ

ABSTRACT

The availability and accessibility of all kinds of data are changing the land-scape of funding, service delivery, and program planning in the human services. For human service organizations to succeed in a quickly changing data landscape, new skills will be required of leaders as well as line staff. This commentary describes the information ecosystem, skills, and training needs of those wishing to thrive in this new world and closes with questions to consider for faculty, students, and administrators in the human services sector.

Introduction

Within a professional lifetime, the nature of social administration has evolved from managing agencies to managing information ecosystems. This metamorphosis will define the nature of what human services managers do and how practice will evolve in the future. Although technology is an important driver of this situation, changes in the political economy, changes in how organizations of all types are managed, and how the social policy enterprise has developed have all played a part in these developments.

In the past, the social work administrator ran an organization. While there were inter-organizational issues to deal with, much of his or her work lay directly within the authority of the position. This changed in the 1960s and 1970s as devolution and contracting took hold (Chalmers & Davis, 2001; Smith & Lipsky, 2009), and many of the agency's activities were managed through contracts rather than directly. Outsourcing and the use of contingent workers also changed the nature of practice. Technology and changes in society are now moving us to the third phase: the virtual economy of care. This will substantially alter the way management of human services organizations is conducted.

The rapidly changing information ecosystem is one example of the quickly evolving digital technology landscape. However, human services leaders are adept at navigating the myriad external forces that shape service delivery. Voida (2011) calls this phenomenon "shapeshifting," suggesting that human service organizations have long histories of adapting to changes across sociopolitical, economic, and technological contexts. Cascio and Montealegre (2016) suggest that new technologies such as cloud computing, artificial intelligence and machine learning, advanced robotics and drones are creating profound changes in how work is done in organizations. These changes are not relegated to the corporate and private sector, and it would be irresponsible for those of us in the nonprofit human services to ignore them.

A substantial body of literature (Cascio & Montealegre, 2016) attests to the fact that technology is an important driver of organizational change. The proliferation of digital technology in the 1980s and 1990s was an important factor leading to smaller, flatter work organizations that engaged in outsourcing and agile production. Although this change has been important in the corporate space, it has also had an effect on public and nonprofit sectors; it has substantially changed management practice and management theory since the 1980s. Technology is important here, but sociocultural and political economy factors are also critical. Many scholars have noted that barriers between sectors have eroded and that communities and external networks have moved from collateral to central positions.

Technology and the rise of information ecologies

From algorithms that can predict academic success and school failure to chatbots that can sort and prioritize clients using natural language processing, the data revolution is undeniably knocking on the door of human services agencies. Although the notions of an information ecology or information ecosystem have been discussed in academic circles since the 1980s, technological developments such as the Internet of Things (IoT), ubiquitous computing, and Big Data have all served to accelerate interest in this arena. Paradoxically, while the data-focused demands on the human services field has increased exponentially over time, commensurate coursework, funding, and professional development preparing social work students and nonprofit leaders for the challenges of the Fourth Revolution, or the management of information ecosystems, has not kept pace. This most recent revolution, still unfolding with the aid of information and communication technologies (ICTs), is turning humans into informational agents in a larger informational ecosystem, and human service organizations intermediaries in the infosphere (Floridi, 2010).[1] Our informational ecosystems may best be understood in terms of informatics, or the application of data collection, analysis, and ICTs to solve problems.

Proposals for a social work informatics have been bandied about on the fringes of the human services world since at least the mid-1990s, if not earlier. Informatics is the science of managing and processing data to transform it into actionable evidence and information (Parker-Oliver & Demiris, 2006; Young, 2000). Informatics and its ally data science have become critical tools for serving professionals in the information marketplace. The goal of social work informatics is to inform decision makers and expand knowledge to deliver efficient, well-managed services (Young, 2000), as in building evidence-based practices, creating evidence-based policies, and other evidence-based decisions.

The adage "knowledge is power" has never been more true and will only continue to exacerbate existing inequalities. We are entering an age of ubiquitous computing, when high levels of social media use, digital personal assistants, and the sensor-embedded physical environments (including public spaces wired with digital cameras, facial recognition software, traffic flow monitors, police listening strategies on social media, and drones, to name just a few) collect digital data about individuals' behavior. In addition, passive data collection about human activities is ceaselessly generated, (Lupton & Williamson, 2017).

While some have described data and its proliferation as the new oil, a persistent divide continues and expands in the digital world, separating what is most recently being called the data-haves and data-have-nots (Gurstein, 2011) or the information-rich and information-poor (Norris, 2003). We could similarly describe the groups as those with data analytic skills versus those without – a variant of the literate versus illiterate in prior periods of history. It is not only a matter of data access but equally importantly, the knowledge and skills for deploying the data to productive purpose. Skills such as data literacy, an understanding of data privacy and security issues and challenges, as well as the opportunities and challenges that these new tools and resources afford organizations, are just a few of the proficiencies required today in a successful human services leader.

---

[1]While a detailed history of ICT in the nonprofit sector is beyond the scope of this editorial, this history may be found in McNutt, Guo, Goldkind, and An (2018). Technology in nonprofit organizations and voluntary action. *Voluntaristics Review, 3*(1), 1–63.

Information ecosystems

Information ecosystems or environments are composed of data generated from client interactions, individuals, organizations, and private corporate data and public data sources such as government agencies at the city, state, and federal level. Public government bodies are among the largest generators and collectors of data in many different domains; one of the key features of this data is that its collection is publicly funded (Janssen, 2011; Janssen, Charalabidis, & Zuiderwijk, 2012). Administrative data is data that derive from the operation of administrative systems, such as tax collection and vital records (Connelly, Playford, Gayle, & Dibben, 2016). Woollard (2014) describes administrative data as information collected for the purposes of registration, transaction, and record keeping, and administrative data are often associated with the delivery of a service. This data may be derived from a broad array of government systems such as housing, transportation, child welfare, and healthcare. Administrative data are a source of large and complex information, and they are considered secondary data that are primarily generated for a purpose other than research. In some nations, such as Norway, Finland, and Sweden, administrative data resources have been available to researchers for many years (see United Nations, 2007). In other parts of the world, especially the United Kingdom and the United States, the recent increased availability of administrative data for research represents a step-change in the social science data infrastructure and a boost for practitioners partnering with academics to investigate how to use data to improve service delivery.

The opening of some of this administrative data is a part of the open data movement, which is still in its infancy. The concept of open data holds significant promise in terms of its potential impact on the human services field, especially regarding the areas of transparency, accountability, and advocacy practices.

Corporate data, or data from the private sector, is proprietary and the property of the companies that collect it. However, implicit data collection – software embedded in the platform economy apps like ride sharing and meal delivery services that collect masses of location data from consumers and drivers – as well as location-based data and health data are also collected from wearable technologies such as fitness trackers or fitness tracking apps and photos and other non-text data such as swipes, gestures, and other movement data that are constantly being captured, collected, and monetized. Data philanthropy, or the idea that corporations can donate these types of unidentified data for the purposes of a social good, is becoming more popular (Taddeo, 2016). Figure 1 depicts a model of information ecosystems in which data from the range of sources can be used by human service providers to improve outcomes for a range of stakeholders.

Changing theoretical frames

The confluence of computing power, available data, ubiquitous computing, and political forces organizing for more transparency and accountability lend themselves to adopting new conceptual models for understanding human service organizations. Complexity theory and collective intelligence are two recent updates to systems theory, a theoretical orientation that social work has historically embraced, which can help human services managers and leaders to make sense of the rapidly changing information ecosystems.

Complexity theory focuses on the study of nonlinear change, a subject that may be all too familiar to our human services professionals. Under a complexity theory orientation, organizations are considered complex adaptive systems (CAS) with characteristics such as interdependence, co-evolution, complexity, and self-organization. However, there is general agreement that a complex system consists of numerous subsystems interacting with each other through multiple, nonlinear, recursive feedback loops (Gilpin & Murphy, 2008).

The complexity of human service organizations and the information ecosystems they may try to navigate is captured by the term *intertwingled*, which refers to the notion that in the real world many systems are connected to each other through those multiple, recursive, nonlinear feedback loops

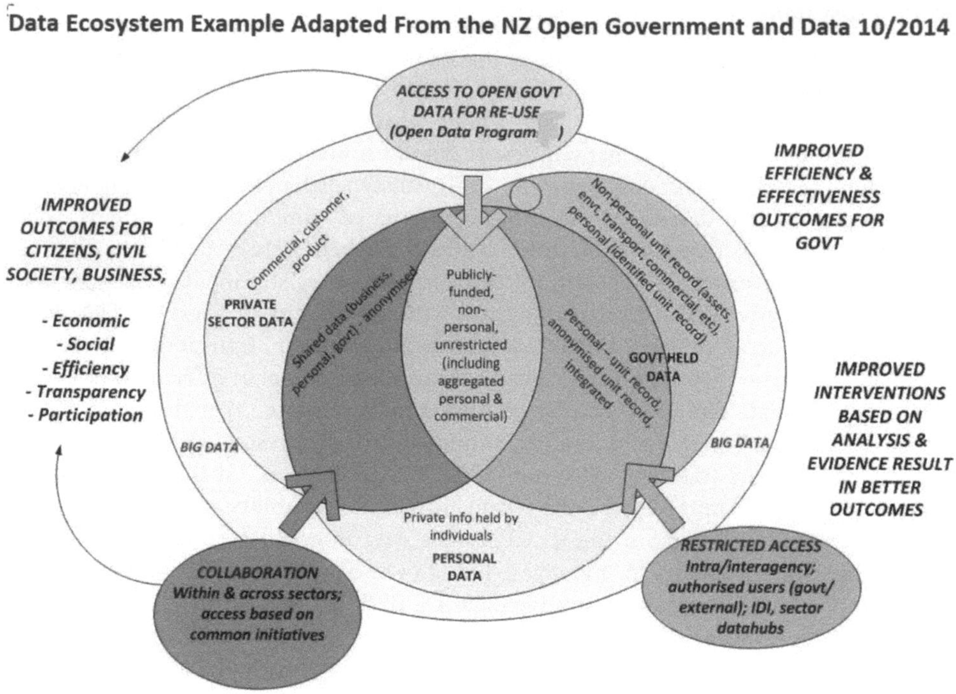

Data Ecosystem Example Adapted From the NZ Open Government and Data 10/2014

Figure 1. Example of an information ecosystem.

(Sanger & Giddings, 2012). The executive director whose programs are funded by multiple agencies collecting comparable but different data on similar outcomes while advocating for new policies for the improvement in access to services for all clients and making a case for service use based on these same data is probably familiar with being interwingled, if not familiar with the exact term.

Similarly, collective intelligence, or the idea of shared or group intelligence that emerges from the collaboration, collective efforts, and competition of many individuals should be familiar to nonprofit human services leaders, at least in principle. Collective intelligence arises as a confluence of collective intelligences (CI), which Levy (2010) broadly defines as "the capacity of human collectives to engage in intellectual cooperation in order to create, innovate and invent" (Levy, 2010, p. 1). While the ideals and philosophy of collective intelligence, especially in organizations, have been germinating since the 1970s, the rise of Web 2.0 networked, cloud-based tools has provided new tools for the support of work flows and structures that may generate collective intelligence. McAfee examined specific opportunities and challenges that Web 2.0 tools can create for organizations (2009), arguing that these tools can be appropriate to support work processes because of three features they present: easy communication and interaction, lack of imposed structure, and mechanisms to let the structures emerge from the community, up into the organization (Matzler, Strobl, & Bailom, 2016).

Changes in technology auger well with many of the changes led by the information society. Technology is clearly part of the "soup" that human service administrators face day to day. In many ways, their evolving role is more planning/organizing and management and less traditional administration. However, the notion that human service administrators must respond to one new technology or even one new social media platform is a red herring; instead, we are suggesting a change in leadership's operational paradigm.

The idea is not about adopting any specific new technology or data collection method; rather, it reflects information and communication environments in which computer sensors (such as radio frequency identification tags and wearable technologies) and hardware (tablets and mobile devices) are unified with other smart objects, people, information, and computers as well as the physical environment (Cascio & Montealegre, 2016). This overall idea is called ubiquitous or pervasive computing. Wooldridge (2015) has called this new world "one that is hyper connected and data saturated, a world where an Internet of everyone is linked to an Internet of everything" (p. 29). Although on its face this may seem daunting, we agree with Voida's assessment (2014) that nonprofits have long histories of adapting to changing circumstances both internal and external to their organizational contexts; ultimately, those that succeed in this information economy will be better equipped to meet and represent the needs of clients and community stakeholders across a range of audiences.

Skills for practice in the information economy

Human service organizations are highly adaptive and will need to pivot and shapeshift by acquiring new organizational skills while enhancing their core community organization and stakeholder management skills to fit the information environment. Below we expand on a few selected skills that will support success in the new information economy.

Managing networks and relationships

The phenomenon of networks and key stakeholder relationships is not new, but the advent of digital tools such as social media platform technologies, crowd funding technologies, and other electronic advocacy strategies have made developing ideological and mission-driven connections considerably more difficult to manage. These examples may be found across the philanthropic communities in foundation affinity groups and local government groups as well as human services provider groups.

Peer networks facilitate learning across organizations, highlight new and emerging best practices and research, and enable mutual assistance among peers, allowing for the possibility of collaborative work to emerge. These networks are seen as a way for leaders to work together by sharing and exchanging information, goals, policies, projects, and best practices to increase chances for success across their respective groups (Fontana, 2017). Today, more and more of these networks are facilitated on electronic platforms with community outreach and policy advocacy activities driven by social media.

Social change and parallel institutions

Parallel institutions set up a parallel structure to an existing system that cannot be changed and is not meeting the needs of the community (Hawk & Zand, 2014). The Gray Areas project of the Ford Foundation promoted their use in America's urban areas in the 1960s (Marris & Rein, 2018), which gave rise to the use of the strategy in the Economic Opportunity Act of 1963, which formulated the Community Action Programs, and later, Community Action Agencies (CAA) as parallel institutions. The rise of alternative social services agencies, such as CAA, free clinics, and radical therapy are examples of the efforts that social workers have created in recent history.

Arising from the work of Gene Sharp, Gandhi, Martin Luther King, Jr. and other scholars of nonviolent civil disobedience, social change and the creation of alternative institutions are based on communities self-organizing to create societal change. One of the key goals of alternative institution building is societal transformation toward a more just and equitable distribution of resources. From Sharp's perspective, a goal of building parallel institutions is to create stronger communal bonds and networks and develop awareness of shared culture, history, and common identities as well as help to frame common grievances, demands, and solutions (Sharp, 1973). This vision is completely consistent with the notion of human service providers as advocates and community conveners when they are representing and standing on behalf of their clients in different social and political situations and before various stakeholders – making presentations before policymakers on behalf of a community, raising awareness and highlighting the concerns of marginalized and underrepresented peoples in popular media platforms (LeRoux, 2014). An example of a parallel institution in the modern domestic U.S. context is the Freedom University in Atlanta, Georgia.

Another relevant parallel institution in the post-modern arena is the use of civic technology in American communities. Civic technology creates new technology infrastructure, sometimes within government and sometimes outside of government (McNutt & Goldkind, 2018). It uses volunteer technologists and engages multiple sectors in creating change.

Virtual organizations are another possibility for parallel institutions and are already represented in significant number in human services. The creation of leaderless, virtual efforts has been part of many emerging political and social movements. Anonymous is one example of a virtual, leaderless organization. Anonymous is a decentralized international hacktivist group that is widely known for its various cyber-attacks against governments, government institutions, and government agencies, nonprofits, and corporations (Fuchs, 2013). Broadly speaking, Anonymous opposes internet censorship and supports internet freedoms. The group's few rules include not disclosing one's identity, not talking about the group, and not attacking media (Olson, 2012).

Social work education for practice in an information economy

While it goes without saying that all social work students, in fact all college graduates, should have a basic understanding of common information and communication technologies and basic data literacy, macro students will need more advanced capacities. Master's-level social workers will operate in a quickly changing and evolving postindustrial society and a virtual economy of care that includes organizations, individuals, and communities. These skills are basic to functioning in a modern organization. Technology has revolutionized education and will continue to grow and develop.

In addition, the following advanced skills are needed:

- Managing organizations in a high-technology environment. This would include a range of skills that include networking, communicating, leveraging power and influence, and so forth; existing curricula could serve as a base for amplifying new environmental factors such as data brokers, social media platforms, and new forms of fundraising. Expanding existing curricula may be less overwhelming for faculty who are unfamiliar with these strategies.
- Managing programs across multiple organizations and networks. This would include techniques in inter-organizational planning and programming, dealing with contracts and agreements, and creating new structures. Curricular content on strategies such as social network analysis, developing collective impact projects, and design thinking would serve to improve student's knowledge and understanding of scenarios for implementing these skills. While inter-organizational practice has always been part of traditional practice, the prospect of many virtual relationships, some transnational in scope, will likely become a part of practice in the future.
- Managing technology projects. This would include planning, budgeting, procurement, and evaluation, and the creation of training and technical support and strategic issues for IT. One can easily imagine existing macro practice and organizationally focused content expanding to include more specified technological content.
- Basic data science and the use of evidence and data in designing program and policy. There are many evidence-based policy-making models and expanding existing policy analysis courses. Existing research courses might be expanded to teach students about data storytelling, data visualization, infographics, and the use of data and evidence to inform a policy brief might make expanding existing curricula less burdensome for instructors.
- Marketing, fundraising, and advocacy in online and offline environments. Here is another place where existing curricula could be enhanced to include more modern and forward-leaning curricula such as electronic fundraising strategies. Similarly, digital advocacy strategies may be included in Community Organizing and Policy courses.

- Advanced networking and the creation of virtual organizations and parallel structures. Similar to the curricular suggestions detailed above, one could imagine existing community organizing curricula to be enhance able to accommodate the inclusion of content on developing virtual organizations and other digital organizing strategies. This is no longer an add-on but represents an important component of social change.

These skills will evolve as society and technology change. Social work and social work education are heading into a new world, not unlike that experienced by the first social workers years ago. As the skills for management in and across information ecologies evolve, the following questions are raised about how service delivery will change:

- How will human service organization leaders use data and information to improve service delivery and develop new services based on data and evidence?
- Who has access to service user data and how do we protect clients and consumers from becoming objectified by their data?
- Where do data literacy and training happen for leaders, line staff, and social work students?
- How can we best help clients navigate these new information ecosystems?

The era of information ecologies offers social work researchers a rich new landscape to partner with human service organizations and scholars in other disciplines. In all areas of human and organizational development, the insertion of new digital tools and tactics raises questions of client/consumer protection and social justice. The scarcity of evidence-based digital interventions in the human services sector opens an exciting area of research opportunities for scholars interested in macro social work and the creation of evidence-informed interventions. The development of new methodologies, and the plentiful data that technology makes available, promises new and exciting research programs.

Future research studies might focus on questions such as:

- What are the training needs of middle managers in order to be successful stewards of information-rich programs?
- How can constituents be incorporated into the management of these new organizations?
- How do emerging technologies change the operation and structure of human services organizations? Will "bricks-and-mortar" organizations predominate in the future or will virtual organizations be the dominant form?
- Will new types of technology assisted fundraising change the relationship between organizations and constituents? Traditional fundraising often led to a preference for large donations from affluent donors. New technology makes fundraising from smaller donors possible because of lower transaction costs.
- How are human service organizations using data science and social informatics in their everyday practice? How can human service organizations create strategic partnerships to gain better access to administrative data? Corporate sector data?
- What is the relationship between online practice and face-to-face practice?
- How are human service organizations prioritizing the education of clients about their data rights and responsibilities and the risks of living in an information society?

These and a myriad of other questions will shape the human services administrative research inquiry for years to come.

Disclosure statement

No potential conflict of interest was reported by the authors.

ORCID

Lauri Goldkind ⓘ http://orcid.org/0000-0002-0967-3960
John G. McNutt ⓘ http://orcid.org/0000-0002-5172-9163

References

Cascio, W. F., & Montealegre, R. (2016). How technology is changing work and organizations. *Annual Review of Organizational Psychology and Organizational Behavior, 3*, 349–375. doi:10.1146/annurev-orgpsych-041015-062352

Chalmers, J., & Davis, G. (2001). Rediscovering implementation: Public sector contracting and human services. *Australian Journal of Public Administration, 60*(2), 74–85. doi:10.1111/ajpa.2001.60.issue-2

Connelly, R., Playford, C. J., Gayle, V., & Dibben, C. (2016). The role of administrative data in the big data revolution in social science research. *Social Science Research, 59*, 1–12. doi:10.1016/j.ssresearch.2016.04.015

Floridi, L. (2010). *Information. A very short introduction.* Oxford, UK: Oxford University Press.

Fontana, F. (2017). City networking in urban strategic planning. In A. Karakitsiou, A. Migdalas, S. T. Rassia, & P. M. Pardalos (Eds.), *City networks: Collaboration and planning for health and sustainability* (pp. 17–38). Cham, Switzerland: Springer.

Fuchs, C. (2013). The Anonymous movement in the context of liberalism and socialism. *Interface: A Journal for and about Social Movements, 5*(2), 345–376.

Gilpin, D. R., & Murphy, P. J. (2008). *Crisis management in a complex world.* New York, NY: Oxford University Press.

Gurstein, M. (2011). A data divide? Data "Haves" and "Have nots" and open (government) data. *Gurstein's Community Informatics.* [Blog post]. Retrieved from https://gurstein.wordpress.com/2011/07/11/a-data-divide-data-%E2%80%9Chaves%E2%80%9D-and-%E2%80%9Chave-nots%E2%80%9D-and-open-government-data/

Hawk, T. F., & Zand, D. E. (2014). Parallel organization: Policy formulation, learning, and interdivision integration. *The Journal of Applied Behavioral Science, 50*(3), 307–336. doi:10.1177/0021886313509276

Janssen, K. (2011). The influence of the PSI directive on open government data: An overview of recent developments. *Government Information Quarterly, 28*(4), 446–456. doi:10.1016/j.giq.2011.01.004

Janssen, M., Charalabidis, Y., & Zuiderwijk, A. (2012). Benefits, adoption barriers and myths of open data and open government. *Information Systems Management, 29*(4), 258–268. doi:10.1080/10580530.2012.716740

LeRoux, K. (2014). Social justice and the role of nonprofit human service organizations in amplifying client voice. In M. J. Austin (Ed.), *Social justice and social work: Rediscovering a core value of the profession* (pp. 325–338). Thousand Oaks, CA: Sage.

Levy, P. (2010). From social computing to reflexive collective intelligence: The IEML research program. *Information Sciences, 180*(1/2), 71–94. doi:10.1016/j.ins.2009.08.001

Lupton, D., & Williamson, B. (2017). The datafied child: The dataveillance of children and implications for their rights. *New Media & Society, 19*(5), 780–794. doi:10.1177/1461444816686328

Marris, P., & Rein, M. (2018). *Dilemmas of social reform: Poverty and community action in the United States.* Abingdon-on-Thames, England: Routledge.

Matzler, K., Strobl, A., & Bailom, F. (2016). Leadership and the wisdom of crowds: How to tap into the collective intelligence of an organization. *Strategy & Leadership, 44*(1), 30–35. doi:10.1108/SL-06-2015-0049

McAfee, A. (2009). *Enterprise 2.0: New collaborative tools for your organization's toughest challenges.* Boston, MA: Harvard Business Press.

McNutt, J. G., & Goldkind, L. (2018). E-Activism development and growth. In *Encyclopedia of information science and technology* (4th ed., pp. 3569–3578). Hershey, PA: IGI Global.

McNutt, J. G., Guo, C., Goldkind, L., & An, S. (2018). Technology in nonprofit organizations and voluntary action. *Voluntaristics Review, 3*(1), 1–63.

Norris, D. F. (2003). Building the virtual state … or not? A critical appraisal. *Social Science Computer Review, 21*(4), 417–424. doi:10.1177/0894439303256728

Olson, P. (2012). *We are Anonymous: Inside the hacker world of LulzSec, Anonymous, and the global cyber insurgency.* New York, NY: Hachette Digital.

Parker-Oliver, D., & Demiris, G. (2006). Social work informatics: A new specialty. *Social Work, 51*(2), 127–134. doi:10.1093/sw/51.2.127

Sanger, M., & Giddings, M. M. (2012). A simple approach to complexity theory. *Journal of Social Work Education, 48*(2), 369–376. doi:10.5175/JSWE.2012.201000025

Sharp, G. (1973). *The politics of nonviolent action.* Boston, MA: Porter Sargent.

Smith, S. R., & Lipsky, M. (2009). *Nonprofits for hire: The welfare state in the age of contracting.* Cambridge, MA: Harvard University Press.

Taddeo, M. (2016). Just information warfare. *Topoi, 35*(1), 213–224. doi:10.1007/s11245-014-9245-8

United Nations. (2007). Register-based statistics in the Nordic countries. In *Review of best practices with focus on population and social statistics* (p. 10). New York, NY: Author.

Voida, A. (2011). Shapeshifters in the voluntary sector: Exploring the human-centered-computing challenges of nonprofit organizations. *Interactions*, *18*(6), 27–31. doi:10.1145/2029976

Voida, A. (2014). A case for philanthropic informatics. In S. Saeed (Ed.), *User-centric technology design for nonprofit and civic engagements* (pp. 3–13). Cham, Switzerland: Springer.

Wooldridge, A. (2015). The Icarus syndrome meets the wearable revolution. In *Korn/Ferry Briefings on Talent and Leadership* (pp. 27–33). New York, NY.

Woollard, M. (2014). Administrative data: Problems and benefits. A perspective from the United Kingdom. In A. Dușa, D. Nelle, G. Stock, & G. Wagner (Eds.), *Facing the future: European research infrastructures for the humanities and social sciences* (p. 35). Berlin, Germany: SCIVERO.

Young, K. M. (2000). *Informatics for healthcare professionals*. Philadelphia, PA: F. A. Davis.

Modest Challenges for the Fields of Human Service Administration and Social Policy Research and Practice

Richard Hoefer

ABSTRACT

Four "Modest Challenges" of importance to scholars and practitioners in human service administration and social policy research are identified and discussed. They are: (1) to more completely identify competencies for social work administration and social policy and which do not acknowledge their dual natures; (2) promote engagement and inclusivity in human service organizations; (3) improve human service pay and equity: and (4) decide whether to engage in advocacy or not. Suggestions for solving these modest challenges include broadening our concepts of both administration and social policy with additional related competencies and concomitant changes in social work curriculum; moving toward a strong inclusivity paradigm within social work practice and academia; supporting NASW efforts for higher pay and greater equity; and aggressively embracing the skills and mindset of advocacy. Successfully addressing these modest challenges lays the foundation for more effective organizations and greater opportunities to solve grander challenges.

A fad has blossomed in recent years – the creation of "Grand Challenges". Poppowitz and Dorgelo (2018) report Grand Challenges are "increasingly being pursued by organizations and individuals" and state "nearly 20 North American universities" (p. 1) were leading such efforts as of October 5, 2017. Weiss and Khaderman (2019) note less than 2 years later that 25 universities in the American Association of Universities and "dozens of other research institutions" have adopted Grand Challenges. The idea is at least a century old and started with mathematics (Global Grand Challenges, n.d., "About Grand Challenges") but the last decade has seen an increase in the number and scope of Grand Challenges efforts. The Bill and Melissa Gates Foundation announced its Global Grand Challenges for Health in 2003 (Global Grand Challenges, n.d., "About Grand Challenges"). On April 2, 2013, the Obama Administration promulgated 21 Grand Challenges to, among other things, "Help tackle important problems related to energy, health, education, the environment, national security, and global development" (Office of Science and Technology Policy, n.d.). Motivations for designating challenges are to spur innovation regarding significant problems and to mobilize hefty resources to tackle them, including developing cross-disciplinary and multi-professional solutions.

Individual professions are involved, as well. In 2008, the National Academy of Engineering announced "14 game-changing goals for improving life on the planet" (National Academy of Engineering, 2008). Social work also has jumped onto the Grand Challenges bandwagon. In 2012, the American Academy of Social Work and Social Welfare (AASWSW) began "to identify 'ambitious yet achievable goals for society" (Padilla & Fong, 2016, p. 133). In the words of AASWSW (n.d.), a Grand Challenge is "a deeply significant problem widely recognized by the public whose solution is within our grasp in the next decade, given concentrated scientific and practical attention" (cited by

Padilla & Fong, 2016, p. 133). Some authors express skepticism over how social work is using Grand Challenges, claiming, for example, that social work's Grand Challenges are neither solvable in the near future (Popple, 2019) nor is the field using the right approaches (Rodriguez, Ostrow, & Kemp, 2016). Yet, support for the idea seems stronger than skepticism.

The challenges identified in this paper for human service organization (HSO) and social policy studies may not be as significant, nor as widely recognized by the public, as other organizations' challenges. It may also be that solutions to these challenges are not within our grasp, as these challenges have existed for decades. Nonetheless, were we to make progress in understanding the modest challenges discussed in this paper, solutions may be closer than they appear at the current time and the contribution to addressing Grand Challenges would be significant.

The Modest Challenges identified here are:

(1) Identifying competencies for social work administration and social policy
(2) Promoting engagement and inclusivity
(3) Improving human services pay and equity
(4) Deciding to engage in advocacy or not

By calling these challenges "modest" rather than "grand", I do not mean to denigrate their importance to researchers and practitioners seeking to understand social work administration and social policy practice. The identified modest challenges are not on the same level as "ensuring healthy development for all youth", or ending homelessness, for example, two of AASWSW's 12 Grand Challenges. Still, successfully addressing these modest challenges lays the foundation for more effective organizations and greater opportunities to solve grander challenges.

Identifying competencies for social work administration and social policy practice

Competencies for administrators have been discussed for decades. An early treatment of the subject titled "The Quest for Competence in Welfare Administration" (Kidneigh, 1950) concludes that it is nearly impossible to agree on a definition of what competence in the field means.

The topic of "competency" is important because social work educators, employers of graduates, and the graduates themselves want to believe that the skills they learn – while in school and/or through other training experiences – will equip them to work effectively and efficiently within the expected parameters of their profession. The National Association of Social Workers Code of Ethics specifically calls for practitioners to "provide services and represent themselves as competent only within the boundaries of their education, training, license, certification, consultation received, supervised experience, or other relevant professional experience" (National Association of Social Workers [NASW], 2017, Section 1.04: Competence). Without clear agreement regarding what competence is for social workers in these roles, it can be easy to run afoul of this ethical standard.

At first glance, it seems that the social work profession has made significant strides in clearly defining what is considered a competency in administrative and social policy practice. Austin (2018) provides a comprehensive history of social work management practice scholarship. Austin et al. (2011) and Hoefer and Sliva (2014) report conducting training programs that included lists of desirable competencies for human service leaders. Peters (2017) provides a new definition of social work leadership. This definition has a validated measure, which connects to needed competencies (Peters & Hopkins, 2019). The *Specialized Practice Curricular Guide for Macro Social Work Practice* (Council on Social Work Education [CSWE], 2018) presents the underlying principles of competency-based education. Competency in social work practice is defined as "the ability to integrate and apply social work knowledge, values, and skills to practice situations in a purposeful, intentional, and professional manner to promote human and community well-being" (CSWE, 2018, p. xv).

More specifically, social workers in administrative practice need to become competent in (at least) these skills: "leadership behaviors, performance management, organizational behavior, evidence-based or promising practices, finances, and budgeting and know how these features of organization life interconnect and influence service effectiveness and talent management" (CSWE, 2018, p. xxviii). Social workers in policy practice should be able to: "shape and affect broad social systems and institutions where laws, regulations, policies, and other wide-ranging decisions that affect human well-being are made", influence "the policy-making process of local, state, and national levels of government, in the executive, legislative, and judicial branches, and in electoral politics," and "amplify the voices and perspectives of marginalized populations within the political arena" (CSWE, 2018, p. xxix).

The Network for Social Work Management (NSWM, 2018) provides another effort to define competencies for human service management. The NSWM document's intent is to specify and detail the competencies with performance indicators necessary to successfully manage human service organizations through the following four domains: Executive Leadership, Resource Management, Strategic Management and Community Collaboration (NSWM, 2018, p. 2). NSWM's work overlaps and dovetails with CSWE's, although it is not identical.

These two lists of competencies seem well-stated and have considerable support. Yet, it is important to acknowledge that every set of competencies has an underlying foundation in a vision of the field the competencies are embedded in. This is not acknowledged by the competency list developers. No list of competencies is "value-neutral".

One of the reasons why defining competencies for administration and social policy is difficult is because the fields both suffer from at least one major division. Each field shows a duality in conceptualization that increases the difficulties in creating definitive lists of competencies.

The duality of administrative practice

Several authors assert that the field of social work/nonprofit administration has a dual nature. Frumkin (2002) labels the two approaches as the "expressive" and the "instrumental" roles of nonprofit management. In a similar vein, Worth (2019) argues that nonprofit human service managers are most often seen in one of two ways. The first view is that of stewards of the public trust and protectors of the civic values embodied in nonprofit organizations (Frumkin's "expressive" dimension). The second is that of managers applying business-related skills to ensure the efficient creation of desired outcomes (p. 13) (Frumkin's "instrumental" dimension). In this regard, the duality may be seen as a social work application of the idea expressed by Bennis and Nanus (2007): "Managers do things right, while leaders do the right things" (p. 12). This can perhaps be rephrased as: Managers engage in instrumental work, while leaders engage in expressive work.

Hasenfeld (2015) argues that social work administration is currently haunted by an inherent contradiction that can be seen as another way to view this "expressive" versus "instrumental" dichotomy. On the one hand, leaders are "expected to embrace values that enhance human dignity, counter discrimination and social stigma, and offer services to reduce suffering and social inequality" (Hasenfeld, p. 1). Yet at the same time, neoliberal processes are designed "to optimize productivity, increase the volume and speed by which clients are processed, reduce costs, and achieve prescriptive performance measures imposed on the workers by top managers (Hasenfeld, p. 2). These two logics are antithetical, according to Hasenfeld. He argues that the dilemma can only be mitigated by (in my terms) managers becoming leaders willing to advocate for values opposing the neoliberal paradigm. Hasenfeld argues that this is a structural situation that impacts individuals serving in those roles.

At its core, different perspectives regarding what the field is lead to different prescriptions for defining competency in social work leadership and management studies. The competencies needed to put forward the expressive side of the field include a thorough grounding in democratic theory, philosophy, economics, religious traditions, and even rhetoric and debate. The expressive position does not talk about return on investment in a monetary sense, although its proponents can argue that helping and educating people improves society as we value each person in a spiritual or humanistic manner.

Instrumentalists want to have a different set of competencies, more akin to what the Council on Social Work Education (2018) and the Network for Social Work Management (2018) propose. While lip service may be paid to the philosophical underpinnings of the nonprofit or human service sectors, the emphasis is undoubtedly on the skills similar to business degree requirements, possibly summed up in the aphorism "There's no mission without money".

The duality of social policy practice

Two subfields of social policy practice exist as well. The older tradition (still well represented in recent work) looks primarily at the history and/or effectiveness of policies. Allen, Garfinkel, and Waldfogel (2018) take this approach as they present a history of social policy research primarily in three arenas: anti-poverty policy, child welfare policy, and health and behavioral health policy. The Social Work Policy Institute (n.d.) follows suit as it provides a list of policy research purposes that seems prescriptive as much as descriptive:

- Assess the needs and resources of people in their environments
- Evaluate the effectiveness of social work services in meeting peoples' needs
- Demonstrate relative costs and benefits of social work services
- Advance professional education in light of changing contexts for practice
- Understand the impact of legislation and social policy on the clients and communities we serve

Allen et al.'s (2018) top-down conceptualization of social policy practice and research is challenged by looking at the purposes of the field from a different view. The second approach focuses the field of social policy on the idea of "policy practice" and "advocacy". Jansson's early (1990) and consistent later work inspired others (Ezell, 2001; Hoefer, 2006, 2019; Rocha, 2007; Schneider & Lester, 2001) to follow in his footsteps of developing policy or advocacy practice as a field. The hallmark of the advocacy practice approach is to ask many more questions regarding "*how*" policy is made, drawing upon the political science literature on legislative processes (including lobbying at all levels of government), interest group activities, administrative practices, and so on.

Just as with the human service administration field, progress toward finalizing competencies in the field of social policy is hampered by a lack of clarity regarding what the key aspects of the field are. If we conceptualize the field of social policy as being mainly about researching policies and their effects (as Allen et al. (2018) reflect), then high levels of research skills are vital. This includes how to find funding for and run complex randomized control-group trial experiments as well as use observational research methods with advanced statistical controls (e.g., panel studies of individual behavior in relation to changes in policies or programs). The ability to analyze data and discuss results, and even disseminate findings to decision-makers, are key in this process as well. These skills are not likely to be widely distributed outside of a few large, elite institutions; instead, they are likely to be relegated to people with advanced degrees and a long apprenticeship with current researchers at those institutions (mostly universities but also consultancies and think-tanks).

If the field of social policy is thought of with a policy practice perspective – that is, advocacy and influencing policy through lobbying, monitoring the administration of laws, affecting budgets, and intervening in court cases – then we must move in another direction. This second path is more amenable to a civic education process and widespread dissemination of how policy practice is conducted. More people can (and must be) involved and motivated to act to have enough influence to counteract the ability of large amounts of funding to sway elected office-holders. (This formulation of the field of social policy as advocacy overlaps significantly with the third macro field, community organizing – an overlap that is unexplored in this manuscript due to space limitations.)

How can human service organizations promote engagement and inclusivity?

One vital aspect of administrative and policy practice is the need to engage with stakeholder groups (such as board members, employees, clients, policy-makers, outside advocates, and funders, among others) who have a range of opinions, different levels of power, and interest in the topics important to social workers and nonprofit organizations. Coalition-building and negotiations take place in various guises in any human service organization or movement. A key skill for all practitioners in the field continues to be the ability to promote engagement so that many voices are represented and to ensure inclusivity of these viewpoints at all stages of decision-making.

According to the latest Gallup study of the situation, the percent of employees in all organizations who consider themselves "engaged" at work (meaning they are "involved in, enthusiastic about, and committed to their workplace") is 34 percent (Gallup, 2018). Nearly one in eight (13%) is "actively disengaged" and over half (53%) are "not engaged". (These percentages actually represent improvement over the past few years.) Gallup argues that their data show that organizations with higher levels of engagement perform at higher levels. Human service organizations may not exactly match these averages but little reason exists to believe that the proportion of workers in the various categories of engagement is much different. It is a waste of resources on a nearly unfathomable level when so many social problems exist. To not have employees fully engaged is an opportunity cost of the highest order.

Inclusivity is related to engagement but goes even further. Mor Barak (2014, 2015) and Mor Barak et al. (2016) provide a useful overview of progress made in this area, particularly in moving beyond the concept of "diversity" to that of "inclusion" in the arena of employment practices. Diversity, she says, is about both observable and non-observable demographic characteristics, while inclusion relates to "employee perceptions that their unique contribution to the organization is appreciated and their full participation is encouraged" (Mor Barak, 2014, p. 85). Mor Barak (2015) provides a clear strategy for promoting inclusion that has both reactive and proactive elements. The process has transformative results when it takes hold: "The inclusive workplace is an action-oriented model for integration of organizations with society via expanding circles of inclusion … to promote inclusion of diversity groups that may not be represented in the organization's workforce" (p. 87). No one believes that making this transition is easy, though the benefits to the organization's employees, clients, community, and beyond are surely worth the effort (Mor Barak et al., 2016).

The issue of inclusivity is often presented as an administrative practice issue. Yet in the same way that diversity and inclusion benefit many elements of the management of human service organizations, they are beneficial in the arena of social policy. For example, much of social policy research focuses on the effectiveness of programs and initiatives that address problems faced by vulnerable and marginalized populations. Increasing diversity and inclusivity of groups not typically involved in social policy research and advocacy would bring relevant experiences and fresh insights to the enterprise. Some approaches to research lend themselves more easily to inclusivity than others and may need to be included (if not privileged) as social policy research is conceptualized and commissioned. One such approach is Community-based Participatory Research (CBPR). As the National Institute on Minority Health and Health Disparities explains, "The community is involved in the CBPR program as an equal partner with the scientists. This helps ensure that interventions created are responsive to the community's needs" (National Institute on Minority Health and Health Disparities, 2018, "Program Description"). Overall, for policy practice adherents as well as human service managers, greater attention to engagement and inclusion may lead to a broader base of ideas and more people working together to bring better results for their activities.

How can human service pay and pay equity be increased?

Social workers' pay and pay equity were discussed over seven decades ago. Wright (1947) finds that many graduates of the School of Social Service Administration at the University of Chicago had done well in their careers. Still, she notes that low pay in general is a problem and that men are paid considerably more than women (Wright, 1947, p. 330).

In naming this topic as a modest challenge, we immediately encounter problems in conceptualizing the issue. Are social work salaries *really* low, and, as compared to what? What variables are associated with different levels of salaries? Given resource constraints and turnover rates, what can be done? These questions are of clear importance to recruiting and keeping capable social workers in the profession at all levels of organizations. Having highly qualified social workers leave the field because pay levels are low is a loss to society and clients who deserve capable staff and effective organizations.

Adding urgency to this challenge is the link with inclusion and equity in human service organizations and the social work research sphere (which is generally situated in academic institutions). Most social work Ph.D. students and future researchers are pulled from the pool of BSW and MSW students who have been in practice, if only because CSWE strongly urges social work programs to have faculty with social work practice experience to teach practice courses, such as administration and policy practice. Thus, we should understand that the context of social work research is predicated on attracting capable students to study social work in the first place. One of the criteria that people use to select their field of work is their ability to earn sufficient income and to be compensated fairly compared to others in the field. Thus, ensuring good and equal pay for social workers in practice has a clear, if indirect, impact on who conducts research on human service organizations and social policy. We should thus be mindful of the long-range implications for social work academia in the pay levels and equity within social work practice.

Empirical wage studies can tell us what actual pay levels are and how they are distributed. Salsberg et al. (2017) have considerable data from which to draw conclusions, though they caution that their public-access data sources do not include everyone with social work education or who work in "social work jobs". Of those employed in social work, many have no social work education or training beyond what is provided on-the-job. Thus, Salsberg and colleagues advise readers to keep data limits in mind as the results are read (p. 4).

Different data sources provide differing answers to the question of compensation levels of people working in social work jobs with at least a bachelor's degree (not necessarily in social work). (All information in this section is from Salsberg et al., 2017.) The Bureau of Labor Statistics (BLS) estimates a median income for social workers of $46,890 in 2016, which is "far less" than for nurses or teachers (p. 6). The American Community Survey (ACS) provides a lower figure: $40,000 in 2015.

Variables that have significant effects on social work compensation include sex, educational level, and job setting. According to ACS data, the median wage for men is $4,000 more per year than for women ($44,000 for men; $40,000 for women) (Salsberg et al., 2017, p. 22, and Table 16, p. 23). Workers with a Bachelor's degree (not necessarily in social work) earn a median wage ($37,000) that is $11,000 less than workers with a Master's degree ($48,000) (again, not necessarily in social work). Having a Ph.D. bumps up the median compensation to $65,000 ($12,000 more than having a Master's degree and $23,000 more than a Bachelor's degree) (Salsberg, et al., p. 23 and Table 17).

Examining the effects of sex and education shows that the disadvantage of being female continue across Bachelor's, Master's, and Ph.D. levels of education (Salsberg et al., 2017, pp. 22–23 and Table 19). Indeed, the percentage of disparity increases as education level rises. At the Bachelor's level, the median income for women is about 8 percent lower than for men ($36,000 to $39,000). At the Master's level, women's median income compared to men is about 12 percent lower ($46,000 compared to $51,500). At the Ph.D. educational level, women's median income is $55,500 while men's is $72,000, a difference of almost 30 percent (Salsberg, et al., pp. 22–23 and Table 19).

Clearly, this information primarily focuses on social workers in practice, with little information concerning researchers. Tower, Faul, Chiarelli-Helminiak, and Hodge (2019) provide recent detailed information concerning the status of women in social work academic settings. Using multivariate analytical techniques with cross-sectional data, Tower and colleagues find that individual characteristics, along with structural ones, are important in understanding why women are paid less than men in social work education. Being employed in a graduate-only program leads to higher salaries compared to teaching in undergraduate-only programs; but in either case, men are paid more than women (p. 361). Women are worse off than men in other characteristics of university life, as well. Women perceive climate factors as more difficult on campuses than do men. Examples include work/life climate, gender equity, sexual harassment, and other forms of discrimination. Women feel more exhausted than men, as well (Tower et al., 2019). As the authors (2019) note drily, "We are clearly not "post-women's equity" (p. 360).

We need to recall that the individuals who are in an academic field in many ways determine what is researched. This is one reason to be concerned with being inclusive across many different identities of applicants for social work academic positions. Research shows that social work education is not replacing the numbers of retiring faculty with new Ph.D. graduates (CSWE, 2016). In many places, social work programs may search in vain for competent researchers interested in policy and administrative practice. This clearly has a detrimental impact on the vigor and even viability of these fields of study.

Should social workers and human service organizations engage in political advocacy?

This seems like a question that may have once been controversial but is now settled. Street's (1931) early social administration text indicates that organizations should conduct advocacy to further their causes. McMillan (1931), in reviewing Street's book, calls for agencies to avoid political advocacy lest the efforts backfire to the detriment of the agency and its clients. One might be forgiven in thinking that the question of social workers and human service organizations being advocates is well settled in the affirmative. The National Association of Social Workers, for example, explicitly endorses social workers being advocates, effectively mandating the practice through its Code of Ethics (NASW, 2017). CSWE (2015) requires students to become competent in advocacy. Some authors (for example, Webster & Abramowitz, 2017) believe the current bitter partisan divide in the United States may require organizations to think again about advocacy work.

The current argument against partisan advocacy (Delaney & Spruill, 2017) is similar to the arguments of the 1930s – i.e., endorsing political positions (and thus, in reality, candidates who support those stands) can lead to negative consequences for the organizations that take them. Donors may flee (although they may also flock), depending on the position taken. Perhaps more worryingly, 501(c)(3) nonprofit organizations may lose their tax-deductible status. The Johnson Amendment (which was authored by then-Senator Lyndon Johnson) was passed in 1954 to prevent nonprofits from endorsing individual candidates for political office. In recent years calls to eliminate it have increased, notably from the Republican party which included the repeal as part of its platform in 2016 (Delaney, 2018). The Republican-controlled U.S. House of Representatives voted three times to eliminate enforcement of the Johnson Amendment in 2017–2018 (Delaney). The argument for eliminating the Johnson Amendment is that it prevents churches from exercising their freedoms of religion and speech. Supporters of current law want to maintain the provision to keep 501(c)(3) organizations from being used to circumvent campaign contribution limits. From a practical perspective, it would be impossible to allow churches and their pastors to speak out and collect funds for specific candidates without also allowing other nonprofits from doing so.

It thus seems that this question of whether to advocate or not has reverted to being controversial when it had not been so for six decades. Yet successful advocacy, led by competent and inspiring social work and human service leaders, may be the only way to achieve progress on the challenges discussed here, including having effective policies, with sufficient funding for those policies and the people who implement them.

How should we address these modest challenges?

Originators of Grand Challenges rarely set about to determine how to meet the challenges themselves. Instead, like Socratic inquiry, challenges encourage the many to develop their own ideas and test them in the open. However, in an effort to spur innovative thinking and action, initial ideas for how to meet the Modest Challenges posed in this paper are outlined here.

Identifying competencies for social work administration and social policy

The changing nature of the fields of practice described here require regular re-visioning of what competencies are needed. We have good ideas regarding competencies for the instrumental view (CSWE, 2018; NSWM, 2018); but scant attention has been paid to the expressive aspect. I suggest that, as the next iteration of review occurs, considerable attention be paid to the "expressive" function of human service organizations and policy practice.

One path toward understanding competencies of expression is to return to some updated version of a classic liberal arts education. Becoming well-versed in philosophy (including theories of government and the nature of civics in relation to humanity) as well as rhetoric and public speaking would allow social workers to engage deeply with and develop their value systems. They would also be able to translate their ideas to others through effective communication strategies.

In addition, administrators and leaders need to understand the importance of emotional intelligence in the form of social and interpersonal skills that are needed for effective and inspiring leadership (Lopes, 2016). Scant attention has been devoted to this topic in the social work literature; and the positive impacts of having these skills might be usefully studied as we seek to understand expressive competencies more fully.

In terms of the duality of ideas regarding social policy, and the competencies each approach needs, we have clear ideas how to teach research methods and statistics. But the lack of a liberal arts-based professional education may lead to technical dexterity with little practical understanding of the values-based implementation and advocacy challenges underlying the policies and programs being researched. Policy practitioners would also benefit greatly from the classic liberal arts foundation background, as ethical clarification and communication skills are beneficial for all. Such courses need to be in Ph. D. coursework requirements as well so that the professoriate can teach the material to their students.

Promoting engagement and inclusivity

Gallup notes that one reason that engagement rates are slowly creeping up may be that managers and supervisors are learning new techniques, such as providing recognition for the positive things employees do and assisting with creating positive relationships between staff members (Gallup, 2018). A return to speaking to everyone in the organization about the ultimate purposes of the organization (beyond a reliance on vision statements or trite motivational posters) may also help with engagement. Most human service workers and policy practitioners have values they want to see enacted – that's why they are in the field. But the burdens of everyday life and work may cause them to lose this fire. Rekindling the spark may reap wonders. A commitment by organizational leaders (at all levels) to implement and sustain shared decision-making can also promote employee engagement that brings positive results (Emerson, Nabatchi, & Balogh, 2012).

Mor Barak (2015) provides a clear strategy for promoting inclusion that has both reactive and proactive elements. The process has transformative results when it takes hold: "The inclusive workplace is an action-oriented model for integration of organizations with society via expanding circles of inclusion … to promote inclusion of diversity groups that may not be represented in the organization's workforce" (p. 87). No one believes that making this transition is easy, though the benefits to the organization's employees, clients, community, and beyond are surely worth the effort (Mor Barak et al., 2016).

Improving human service pay and equity

The National Association of Social Workers is using several strategies to increase social workers' pay. Advocacy is one of the most important (see next topic as well). For example, NASW works to ensure that licensed social workers are hired for certain positions in state government. Further, legislating title protection (only licensed social workers can work in "social worker" jobs) has been a major purpose of NASW advocacy. Advocacy for Medicare reimbursement rate increases is another means to try to increase social workers' incomes. Finally, NASW is developing certification programs in health care to improve social workers' competitiveness in well-paying hospital settings (Wright, 2019). Universities are also moving toward offering certificate programs (such as nonprofit management) for current students to expand their knowledge base. Working professionals may also find skills-enhancing courses and certificates through universities and professional organizations. These programs allow the participants to increase their job skills, regardless of their past degrees. All of these efforts may, in time, lead to a broader and higher paid pool of practice-qualified researchers in administrative and policy practice realms. As Schweitzer, Chianello, and Kothari (2013) remind us, compensation levels in the field of social work are critical for worker satisfaction and for sustaining the profession. This statement presumably applies to those at the Ph.D. level conducting research as well as at the BSW and MSW levels, including those studying macro practice.

Deciding to engage in advocacy or not

Effective advocacy can overcome the current political climate of demonization of immigrants, attacks on policies beneficial to vulnerable populations, and endless war overseas. It also can be used to improve workplaces and public policies regarding pay levels and equal treatment of all. Appeasement is not a viable alternative, nor is hoping that "things will improve on their own". Rather than backing away from advocacy, it is vital to learn more about how to conduct successful advocacy and to teach it well to students. A number of useful texts exist but faculty need to learn more about the topic in order to effectively teach the material (Maleku & Hoefer, 2017; Weiss-Gal, 2016).

Conclusion

The Grand Challenges approach to focusing attention and scholarship on particular topics has value, although a set of modest challenges precedes it. The selection of particular topics is driven by many forces and not everyone will agree on their importance or ordering, regardless of how inclusive the process is. It can be difficult for experts in smaller professional niches to find a way to contribute to Grand Challenges endeavors.

Taking a step back from the largest and most difficult issues of our time to address many Modest Challenges may be the best approach to actually solving the Grand Challenges of social work. Before the United States could send a man to the moon and return him safely – a Grand Challenge of the 1960s, many equally difficult challenges had to be solved, including developing new materials, inventing healthy foodstuffs, creating mathematical approaches, and so on. None of these Modest Challenges were enough, by themselves, to achieve the safe exploration of the moon, but they were necessary steps.

Adopting the tack of naming and overcoming Modest Challenges can lead scholars and practitioners to approach problem solving on a more local and "fixable" level. It is less daunting to discuss the gaps that need filling and to find solutions if the challenges are of smaller proportions. The two small fields of human service administration and social policy are good examples of how the process could work for other subfields. Identifying required competencies for practitioners in these fields advances the ability of organizations to serve clients across all of social work. Increasing engagement and adding inclusion practices positively affect organizational effectiveness in each part of social work. Improving pay levels and decreasing inequities sends ripples throughout the entirety of human services, leading to better recruitment and retention of skilled practitioners and scholars. Adding advocacy skills and using them successfully is the only path to achieving the Grand Challenges laid out for us.

As modest as the challenges discussed in this paper may seem at first glance, they have grand implications for the improvement for research, teaching, and practice for human service organizational and social policy practice. By successfully addressing these modest challenges, we will be able to contribute in a substantial way to improving society and resolving far grander ones.

Acknowledgments

The author would like to acknowledge the sustained support of Bowen McBeath and Karen Hopkins in the development of this manuscript. Genevieve Graff reviewed a late version of the manuscript.

Disclosure statement

No potential conflict of interest was reported by the author.

References

Allen, H., Garfinkel, I., & Waldfogel, J. (2018). Social policy research in social work in the twenty-first century: The state of scholarship and the profession; what is promising and what needs to be done. *Social Service Review*, 92(4), 504–547. doi:10.1086/701198

Austin, M. (2018). Social work management practice, 1917–2017: A history to inform the future. *Social Service Review*, 92(4), 548–616. doi:10.1086/701278

Austin, M., Regan, K., Samples, M., Schwartz, S., & Carnochan, S. (2011). Building managerial and organizational capacity in nonprofit human service organizations through a leadership development program. *Administration in Social Work*, 35(3), 258–281. doi:10.1080/03643107.2011.575339

American Academy of Social Work and Social Welfare (AASWSW) (n.d.). Grand Challenges for Social Work. Retrieved from. http://grandchallengesforsocialwork.org/grand-challenges-initiative/12-challenges/

Bennis, W. G., & Nanus, B. (2007). *Leaders: The strategies for taking charge*. New York, NY: HarperCollins.

Council on Social Work Education. (2016). *Annual statistics on social work educational programs*. Alexandria, VA: Author. Retrieved from https://www.cswe.org/getattachment/992f629c-57cf-4a74-8201-1db7a6fa4667/2015-Statistics-on-Social-Work-Education.aspx

Council on Social Work Education (CSWE). (2015). 2015 Educational policy and accreditation standards for baccalaureate and master's social work programs. Alexandria VA: Council on Social Work Education. Retrieved from. https://www.cswe.org/CSWE/media/AccredidationPDFs/2015-epas-and-glossary_1.pdf

Council on Social Work Education. (2018). *Specialized practice curricular guide for macro social work practice*. Alexandria, VA: Author. Retrieved from https://www.cswe.org/getattachment/Education-Resources/2015-Curricular-Guides/2015-Macro-Guide-Web-Version.pdf.aspx

Delaney, T. (2018, July 24). *Could this political environment get more toxic for nonprofits? The answer is yes unless you act today*. Nonprofit Quarterly. Retrieved from https://nonprofitquarterly.org/johnson-amendment-act-today/

Delaney, T., & Spruill, V. (2017, March 22). Keep partisan politics out of the nonprofit sector. *The Hill*. Retrieved from https://thehill.com/blogs/pundits-blog/the-administration/325126-keep-partisan-politics-out-of-the-nonprofit-sector

Emerson, K., Nabatchi, T., & Balogh, S. (2012). An integrative framework for collaborative governance. *Journal of Public Administration Research and Theory*, 22(1), 1–29. doi:10.1093/jopart/mur011

Ezell, M. (2001). *Advocacy in the human services*. Belmont, CA: Brooks/Cole.

Frumkin, P. (2002). *On being nonprofit: A conceptual and policy primer*. Cambridge, MA: Harvard University Press.

Gallup. (2018, August 26). *Employee engagement on the rise*. Retrieved from https://news.gallup.com/poll/241649/employee-engagement-rise.aspx?utm_source=link_wwwv9&utm_campaign=item_245786&utm_medium=copy

Global Grand Challenges. (n.d.). *About*. Retrieved from https://gcgh.grandchallenges.org/about

Hasenfeld, Y. (2015). Exactly what is human service management? *Human Service Organizations: Management, Leadership, and Governance*, 39(1), 1–5. doi:10.1080/23303131.2015.1007773

Hoefer, R. (2006). *Advocacy practice for social justice*. Chicago, IL: Lyceum Press.

Hoefer, R. (2019). *Advocacy practice for social justice* (4th ed.). New York, NY: Oxford University Press.

Hoefer, R., & Sliva, S. (2014). Assessing and augmenting administration skills in nonprofits: An exploratory mixed methods study. *Human Service Organizations: Management, Leadership, & Governance, 38*(3), 246–257. doi:10.1080/23303131.2014.892049

Jansson, B. (1990). *Social welfare policy: From theory to policy practice.* New York, NY: Brooks/Cole.

Kidneigh, J. C. (1950). The quest for competence in welfare administration. *Social Service Review, 24*(2), 173–180. doi:10.1086/637836

Lopes, P. (2016). Emotional intelligence in organizations: Bridging research and practice. *Emotion Review, 8*(4), 316–321. doi:10.1177/1754073916650496

Maleku, A., & Hoefer, R. (2017). Social work academia and policy in the United States. In J. Gal & I. Weiss-Gal (Eds.), *Where academia and policy meet: A cross-national perspective on the involvement of social work academics in social policy* (pp. 221–241). Bristol, UK: Policy Press.

McMillan, A. (1931). Review of *social work administration. Social Service Review, 5*(4), 670–672. doi:10.1086/630980

Mor Barak, M. E. (2014). *Managing diversity: Toward a globally inclusive workplace* (3rd ed.). Thousand Oaks, CA: Sage.

Mor Barak, M. E. (2015). Inclusion is the key to diversity management, but what is inclusion? *Human Service Organizations: Management, Leadership & Governance, 39*(2), 83–88. doi:10.1080/23303131.2015.1035599

Mor Barak, M. E., Lizano, E, Kim, A., Duan, L., Rhee, K., Hsiao, & Brimhall, K. (2016). The promise of diversity management for climate of inclusion: A state-of-the-art review and meta-analysis. *Human Service Organizations: Management, Leadership & Governance, 40*(4), 305–333. doi:10.1080/23303131.2016.1138915

National Academy of Engineering. (2008). *14 game-changing goals for improving life on the planet.* Retrieved from http://www.engineeringchallenges.org/challenges.aspx

National Association of Social Workers. (2017). *Code of ethics.* Retrieved from https://www.socialworkers.org/About/Ethics/Code-of-Ethics/Code-of-Ethics-English

National Institute on Minority Health and Health Disparities. (2018, October 2). *Program description.* Retrieved from https://www.nimhd.nih.gov/programs/extramural/community-based-participatory.html

Network for Social Work Management. (2018). *Human service management competencies: A guide for nonprofit and for-profit agencies, foundations, and academic institutions.* Retrieved from https://socialworkmanager.org/wp-content/uploads/2018/12/HSMC-Guidebook-December-2018.pdf

Office of Science and Technology Policy. (n.d.). *21st century grand challenges.* Retrieved from https://obamawhite house.archives.gov/administration/eop/ostp/grand-challenges

Padilla, Y., & Fong, D. (2016). Identifying grand challenges facing social work in the next decade: Maximizing social policy engagement. *The Journal of Policy Practice, 15*(3), 133–144. doi:10.1080/15588742.2015.1013238

Peters, C., & Hopkins, K. (2019). Validation of a measure of social work leadership. *Human Service Organizations: Management, Leadership & Governance, 43*(2), 92–110. doi:10.1080/23303131.2019.1606869

Peters, S. C. (2017). Social work leadership: An analysis of historical and contemporary challenges. *Human Service Organizations: Management, Leadership & Governance, 41*(4), 336–345. doi:10.1080/23303131.2017.1302375

Popple, P. (2019). *Grand challenges for social work and society* [Review]. *Social Service Review, 93*(1), 129–133. doi:10.1086/702830

Poppowitz, M., & Dorgelo, C. (2018). *Report on university-led grand challenges.* UCLA: Grand Challenges. Retrieved from https://escholarship.org/uc/item/46f121cr

Rocha, C. (2007). *Essentials of social work policy practice.* Hoboken, NJ: John Wiley & Sons.

Rodriguez, M., Ostrow, L., & Kemp, S. (2016). Scaling up social problems: Strategies for solving social work's grand challenges. *Research on Social Work Practice.* doi:10.1177/1049731516658352

Salsberg, E., Quigley, L., Mehfoud, N., Acquaviva, N., Wych, K., & Sliwa, S. (2017). *Profile of the social work workforce.* Washington, D.C.: George Washington University Health Workforce Institute and School of Nursing. Retrieved from https://www.socialworkers.org/LinkClick.aspx?fileticket=wCttjrHq0gE%3d&portalid=0

Schneider, R., & Lester, L. (2001). *Social work advocacy: A new framework for action.* Belmont, CA: Brooks/Cole.

Schweitzer, D., Chianello, D., & Kothari, B. (2013). Compensation in social work: Critical for satisfaction and a sustainable profession. *Administration in Social Work, 37*(2), 147–157. doi:10.1080/03643107.2012.669335

Social Work Policy Institute. (n.d.). *Why do we need social work research?* Retrieved from http://www.socialworkpolicy.org/research

Street, E. (1931). *Social work administration.* New York, NY: Harper Brothers.

Tower, L., Faul, A., Chiarelli-Helminiak, C., & Hodge, D. (2019). The status of women in social work education: A follow-up study. *Affilia, 34*(3), 346–368. doi:10.1177/0886109919836105

Webster, S., & Abramowitz, A. (2017). The ideological foundations of affective polarization in the U.S. electorate. *American Politics Research, 45*(4), 621–647. doi:10.1177/1532673X17703132

Weiss, J., & Khaderman, A. (2019, September 3). *What universities get right—And wrong—About grand challenges.* Inside Higher Education. Retrieved from https://www.insidehighered.com/views/2019/09/03/analysis-pros-and-cons-universities-grand-challenges-opinion

Weiss-Gal, I. (2016). Policy practice in social work education: A literature review. *International Journal of Social Welfare, 25*, 290–303. doi:10.1111/ijsw.12203

Worth, M. (2019). *Nonprofit management: Principles and practice* (5th ed.). Thousand Oaks, CA: Sage.

Wright, G. (2019, May 2). *What can be done to raise social work salaries?* Retrieved from http://www.socialworkblog. org/pressroom/2019/03/what-can-be-done-to-raise-social-work-salaries-listen-to-our-podcast-series-and-give-us-your-comments/

Wright, H. (1947). Employment of graduates of the school of social service administration. *Social Service Review, 21*(3), 316–330. doi:10.1086/636403

Evaluating Behavioral and Organizational Outcomes of Leadership Development in Human Service Organizations

Karen Hopkins and Megan Meyer

ABSTRACT

The health of the human services sector depends upon equipping both emerging and current leaders with key leadership skills to help them increase their organization's capacity and effectiveness. Yet while most leadership development programs intend that participants will acquire and apply new learning, program assessment tends to focus more on the acquisition of knowledge and skills rather than the application of learning through changed behaviors that lead to desired organizational outcomes. We provide a summary of current leadership development efforts and new orientations, describe the development of a flexible, embedded in practice, human services leadership and management certificate program, and highlight potential and planned strategies for evaluating and measuring change in both individual leaders or a collective group of leaders within or across organizations, and in organizational outcomes, all of which can be replicated and enhanced in future research.

The world of work, the goals we set, and the needs we meet, require we assess the behavioral outcomes and impact of leadership development in human service organizations (HSOs) and enterprises of all sorts. While most educational institutions and current leadership programs intend that participants will acquire and apply new learning, program assessment tends to focus on the acquisition of knowledge rather than the application of knowledge through changed behaviors that lead to desired organizational outcomes. So in the face of emerging new demands for organizational performance improvement, how can we shift to more effectively evaluate leadership development programs and measure behavior change through learning interventions? In this commentary, we summarize what we know about current leadership development efforts and new orientations, describe the development of a flexible, embedded in practice, human services leadership and management certificate program, and we discuss potential and planned strategies for evaluating and measuring behavior change in program participants and organizational outcomes that can be replicated and enhanced in future research.

Leadership development in the human services

Nonprofit and public HSOs desperately need innovative leadership development. Many professionals in HSOs find themselves thrust into managerial and leadership positions without the requisite knowledge and skills necessary to be effective (Austin, 2018; Bernotavicz, McDaniel, Brittain, & Dickinson, 2013; Coloma, Gibson, & Packard, 2012; Rofuth & Piepenbring, 2020; Shera & Bejan, 2017). In turn, many current human service managers recognize their leadership limitations and desire new approaches and leadership skills to help them increase their organization's capacity and effectiveness (Hodges & Howieson, 2017; Hopkins, Meyer, Shera, & Peters, 2014; Rofuth & Piepenbring, 2020). Thus, the health of the human services sector depends upon equipping both emerging and current leaders with key managerial and leadership skills and flexibly meeting leaders' needs at any point along their leadership development path (sometimes referred to as "leader" development), as well as focusing attention on broader shared "collective" learning interventions within and across organizations (sometimes referred to as "leadership" development, i.e., Hanson, 2013).

Educational institutions and organizations have responded to this growing need for "on the job" leader/leadership development, proliferating programs of various sorts, including continuing education certificates and in-house or online training, which continue to evolve to meet the demands of working participants. Other strategies include "lunch and learn" sessions, leadership retreats, conversational coaching with staff, and succession planning (Vito, 2018). Some common elements of desirable leadership development (term herein used) programs for individual participants include enrollment, schedule, and content flexibility (Hassell, 2016; Hopkins, Meyer, Cohen-Callow, Mattocks, & Afkinich, 2019). Nevertheless, despite the influx of online education opportunities, the default posture for learning interventions and programs remains the traditional in-person, instructor-led engagement, with more emphasis on a "banking" form of content delivery rather than real-time application of learning to ongoing challenges leaders face in their organizations. So, in short, we often continue to emphasize the "what" of learning, even as more evidence emerges that suggests "how we learn" is more important (Gino, 2018; Kennedy, Carroll, & Francoeur, 2013; Liedtka, 2018).

For instance, organizations increasingly want more custom-built, agile, applicable, and consultative approaches to learning versus "canned content" (Feser, Nielsen, & Rennie, 2017; Hassell, 2016; Meyer & Hopkins, 2019). Off the shelf curricula are less effective because the nature, speed, and intensity of change mean that organizations and their leaders will be facing more situations that are new and unfamiliar, not only to the leaders themselves but to the organizations as well. This means that organizations seek collaborative engagements with educational institutions, learning providers, and stakeholders to assess individual learning needs, challenges unique to an organization's growth cycle, and to respond with content and learning exposures that align with both the practitioner and organizational objectives (Hassell, 2016).

As organizations face more uncertainty and change, learning strategies shift to focus on developing behaviors that productively manage risk-taking, drive truly inclusive people management, and innovatively design collaborative work to strategically lead organizations to breakthrough performance (The Jensen Group, 2014; Whitney, 2016). In this context, whatever the mechanism, modality, or means of development deployed, the goals of the learning experience shift from knowledge acquisition, per se, toward skill building, behavior change, and mindset – the foundations of lasting and agile development (Hamman & Spayd, 2015). Nevertheless, research suggests that many programs either fail to achieve their goals or cannot successfully measure results beyond attainment of new knowledge (Ardichvilli, Natt och Dag, & Manderscheid, 2016; Feser et al., 2017; Hanson, 2013).

New leadership orientations

Thus, it should come as no surprise that we see new perspectives on leadership development and more innovative approaches to delivering content emerging. For example, embedding learning in workflows in order to demonstrate needed leadership skills and competencies has gained ground. The days of pulling people "from the line", so to speak, to sit in classes or programs for extended periods of time has given way to more work-integrated approaches that offer "just in time" exposure to the right content for the right people. Organizations have also turned from external "expert-delivered" learning to peer-to-peer collaborations that offer relevant knowledge in a work appropriate manner that ensures uptake and adoption (Baker, 2014; Palmer & Blake, 2018).

Additionally, organizations adapt methods to challenge and/or change the "mindset" of individuals or teams in a more relationship-based and immersive approach. This strategy deploys collaborative questioning, team-based hypothesizing, data gathering, testing assumptions and practices, and aligning vision to outcomes related to the nature of the work (Kennedy et al., 2013). It embeds learning as part of work processes and transforms learning from a stand-alone experience to a work-related endeavor whose purpose is to iterate toward continuous adaptation in a changing environment.

Ultimately, both orientations are essential to holistically develop leaders who can take hold of new knowledge and skills and a newly-framed mindset to skillfully steer and navigate complex human service environments. This is where a coaching component to leadership development can help link individual or team learning to the organization's needs and experiences.

Program description

We developed a Human Services Leadership and Management Certificate program at the University of Maryland School of Social Work in response to the rapid growth of the health and human service and non-profit sectors in the last decade. The vision for it is to be a vital and competitive educational and coaching program for human service professionals that expands the capacity of the University of Maryland to meet the future leadership demands of the private and public human services sector. The mission is to develop the leadership and management capacity of alumni and human service professionals in the Baltimore–Washington metro region through flexible, customizable, competency-based education, facilitated peer coaching, and networking.

Initial planning and market assessment

Our work, beginning in 2012, to develop the Human Services Leadership and Management Certificate included: (1) an environmental scan of both existing masters programs in non-profit leadership and leadership certificate programs in the Baltimore–Washington metro region; (2) an assessment of the success factors possessed by the University of Maryland School of Social Work that positioned it to establish a niche and complement existing programs in the region; and (3) interviews with human service agency leaders and directors of other more established leadership development programs. Our scan revealed that the existing programs ranged from 8 to 9-day "boot camps" or certificate cohort models with low price points (approximately $1500) to credit-bearing certificate programs embedded within existing MBA, public policy or arts and sciences masters programs, with much higher price points (from $8,000-$20,000) and requiring admission to and completion of full masters programs. While the programs we examined shared many similarities in purpose and content, none targeted leadership in human service organizations specifically nor offered the flexibility we knew our audience of MSW alumni and other working human service professionals needed at an affordable price point.

Guiding principles and core components

Based upon our environmental scan and assessment of our target audience's needs, we developed a set of guiding principles for our program:

- Competency-based assessment and learning for current and future-oriented leaders.
- Flexible, customizable, in-person, hybrid and on-line program offerings.
- Affordable ($2500) with the added provision of continuing education units (CEUs).
- Embedded and real-time learning, where workshops and facilitated peer coaching are used as critical tools for leadership development among participants currently working in human service organizations.

- A non-cohort "open" model where educational offerings are open to any alumni and human service professional whether they commit to completing the entire certificate program or not.

With these principles in mind, we identified four core components of the certificate:

(1) A competency-based self-assessment designed to help participants determine which leadership skills they may need to improve most; (2) Core content that includes three modules (5 days) on leadership style and building leadership potential, applying coaching to leadership situations, and developing supervisors as leaders; (3) Customizable content (10 one-day modules) where participants can choose from a menu of offerings based on their self-assessment, leadership aspirations and needed skills; and (4) Facilitated peer-coaching circles (six sessions) for at least 1 year during the progression through the certificate. Our requirement of peer coaching is aligned with research that shows learning is facilitated in collaborative settings where knowledge is shared and problems are solved together, whether it be face-to-face or on a platform like Zoom, Skype or Google, etc. (Moldoveanu & Narayandas, 2019).

Piloting and implementing program iterations

We arrived at this (above) version of our certificate program after several years of piloting the core certificate components and learning that we, ourselves, needed to be flexible and adaptable in how these components were implemented. First, we determined our online competency-based assessment tool was too long and complex as participants were not fully completing it and/or contacting us with questions about the instrument. We again researched the literature and implemented a new tool that is more user-friendly and informative for participants' self-assessment. Next, we adjusted our core content, which originally included more required modules, and increased our customizable content (and instructors) each year, as our participants range from newly minted supervisors to more experienced organizational directors with different learning needs and aspirations. Finally, we adjusted the number of facilitated peer-coaching circle sessions from 10 to 6 as the professional coaches determined, after several years, that learning application saturation was occurring among the participants within six coaching sessions.

With these adjustments, participants are able to complete the program within 18 months, but are allowed to take multiple years and proceed at a pace that is most useful to them. While cohort models can provide a high-intensity experience and significant relationship building and bonding among a group, the downside of cohort models is that participants return to their workplaces without follow-up and support for embedded application of the knowledge and skills they gained in training. Our model captures the bonding benefits that result from cohort models with the required peer-coaching component of the program without forcing participants to find the time to commit to a pre-set 1–2 (or more) week cohort model. Our model also creates an iterative experience for participants, where they can practice applying their learning and then process the challenges they experienced among a peer group, and adjust their future practice accordingly. This model shifts learning toward the state-of-the-art skill building, behavior change, and mindset approach described earlier as critical by other leadership development scholars (Hamman & Spayd, 2015).

Taking the time to pilot the leadership certificate program provided us the opportunity to gradually implement the structural and procedural changes needed to improve the program components and build a base of participants. Now we are at the stage of both developing and implementing an evolving evaluation plan, but will it be the most effective evaluation model for assessing and documenting the outcomes and impact of our leadership development efforts? This question, which plagues so many researchers and management practitioners, is what drives our commentary. To flesh this out for both human service organization researchers and managers, we propose a combination of our ideas and evaluation plan, including a smattering of what we know has worked or been tried by others, and what we believe has the potential to deliver the kind of results or findings that have eluded the leadership field.

Measuring the outcomes of leadership development

Traditional methods of assessing outcomes of leadership development, such as individual structured evaluations and pre-post competency assessments, are not enough to adequately capture whether the learning is embedded and implemented effectively within the organizational context (Edwards & Turnbull, 2013; Feser et al., 2017); thus, requiring assessment to bridge between individual or team learning and the impact on mindset, performance, and the organization.

Are we asking the right evaluative questions?

Ideally, the questions and measures for evaluating learning and performance development should reflect a balance between the individual learners and the workforce and workplace, including potential funders that may be financing the learning process. In fact, the individual-team-organizational connection has to begin before the learning development proceeds. For example, what is the individual/team and organizational rationale for leadership development and what are the expectations post-development? Who is or should be part of this discussion? Leadership development needs to be grounded in the organizational context of service demands and account-ability. Thus, what is expected to be the return on investment (ROI) as a result of leadership development – simply individual leadership skill acquisition or different or transformed processes within the organization or in services to its community or constituents?

Additionally, often the effects of leadership learning do not occur immediately and need to be assessed over time to reduce the underestimation of results (Fisher, Dietz, & Antonakis, 2016). Taking a more longitudinal perspective, we envision leadership development evaluation on a continuum from *individual* assessment and learning application to *collective group/team* assessment of behavior change to assessment of *organizational program or team performance* (see Figure 1). First assessing, *What did the individual learner gain in knowledge, skills, vision, and ideas for further action?* Next, after an appropriate period of time depending on the type of learning, asking, *How specifically did that learning get implemented in the organization?* Then, following up later, *How impactful was the learning on the workforce and the work itself?* For example, *How did the learning help address the organization's talent and performance management needs? What program or*

Individual			Collective Group/Team		Organization	
Pre and post self-assessment - knowledge -skills -behaviors	Personal learning and action plans for transfer of learning Participant journaling of successes and challenges in transfer of learning	360 degree evaluations by agency members (facilitated by coaches)	Peer circle coach assessment of learning application, behavior change, and outcomes Peer circle coach assessment of benefits of coaching to group/ sector overall	Focus groups or interviews with participants about experiences with learning, coaching, application, behavior changes, and team/ organization outcomes	Surveys and interviews with managers to corroborate transfer of learning to organization impact Participant journaling about impact of transfer of learning on organization or service performance	Assessment of changes in team or program performance data, and/or organization changes Assessment of alignment of leadership development interventions and organization efforts to sustain changes

Figure 1. Continuum of leadership development evaluation.

organizational transformations were initiated? When organizations or funders choose to provide/pay for leadership development, they increasingly want to know what competitive advantage their grantees or grantee sector gain as a result (Whitney, 2016). *How beneficial is leadership development and learning to the organization (and even the HSO sector in a particular field or geographic area)? How has leadership development helped the organization(s) to succeed? Is it worth the investment?*

What are the evaluation strategies to consider?

Individual assessment

Individual evaluation strategies that are part of our evolving evaluation plan include: 1) examining pre- and post-learning assessments to track knowledge and skills gained, and in what content areas, 2) having participants complete an action plan detailing how they intend to incorporate and transfer key components of their learning to the work setting, and 3) regular conversations with coaches which will provide ongoing information about individual growth and application of learning. Examples of participants' action plans include "Personal Learning" or "Change Initiative" plans (Bernotavicz et al., 2013), and a "Learning Resume and Experience Plan", which require individuals to meet with managers (or team members) prior to training sessions to prioritize learning skills and identify upcoming practice opportunities and experiences within the organization so that participants become more purposeful in how they learn (Roberts, 2015). Additionally, post-training assignments or homework in-between ongoing learning and coaching sessions that get reviewed by training facilitators, coaches, and/or organizational managers helps both reinforce and track learning outcomes (Austin, Regan, Samples, Schwartz, & Carnochan, 2011; Shera & Bejan, 2017). Thus, a key strategy for tracking individual leadership development outcomes lies in some form of a written goal-setting and action plan for learning transfer, ideally designed through a development conversation between the participants and their manager or team, prior to learning and coaching sessions.

This type of plan provides a mechanism by which learning facilitators, coaches, and evaluators/researchers can follow-up with participants to assess the results or impact of learning development within their organizations over time. Managers and team members can also continue to benefit from such a plan by having ongoing professional development conversations with their employees/peers, including development check-ins for performance guidance and support.

Coaches are critical conduits in "evidence gathering" in our evaluation plan, such as evaluating participants in their application and implementation of learning – knowledge, skills, and leadership mindset – throughout each coaching session and over time. Coaches determine and track, *What is the most important problem the learner wants to solve, how does the learner approach it, who does the learner involve, and what is the result?* Potentially as part of the coaching process, coaches can be actively involved in collecting 360-degree evaluation data from appropriate organizational members for each participant, as piloted by Coloma et al. (2012) with a cohort of public human service managers.

Our experience with the required peer-coaching component of our program and feedback from participants shows how meaningful this type of coaching is, especially for young women identified as "rising stars", and human service professionals of color who tend to get less mentoring than men and whites, and who are very underrepresented in leadership roles. Other feedback we have received demonstrates participants' enthusiasm in "taking back" and sharing concepts, ideas, and exercises from the learning and coaching with their organizational members, board, and other partners. The reinforcement of learning, support, and career development contributes to the application of leadership learning and builds capacity for management roles (Hopkins et al., 2019; Meyer & Hopkins, 2019).

Collective group/team assessment

While coaching in a variety of forms, including facilitated peer circle coaching (an important component of our certificate program), has grown as a key component of leadership programs to help participants move from learning to action, there is little empirical evidence demonstrating the impact of coaching on team and organizational performance (Beattie et al., 2014). Thus, a key question is, *How effective is coaching in facilitating learning implementation and solving real organizational or service delivery problems?*

We are currently experimenting with two models of peer learning and coaching that has the potential to influence the capacity of an entire group/team, beyond individual participant gains. One involves a large well-reputed human service agency with multiple satellite offices across Baltimore City, which has enrolled their 17 program and site managers in the leadership certificate and coaching program. As the managers progress through the leadership learning content, they are also participating in facilitated peer-coaching circle sessions with a certified coach to focus on application of learning content specific to *one* organization's work. The second model involves collaboration with a long-standing and highly regarded local Foundation to provide organizational and leadership development and facilitated peer coaching to the directors/managers of nonprofit agency grantees across five neighborhoods in Baltimore City.

The participants in both of these models are collectively (across an organization and across a sector with a common funder) building their leadership skills, and through coaching figuring out *together* how to apply the learning for greater organizational and community impact. This kind of collective leadership development not only lends itself to sharing knowledge and information and innovative ideas for wider benefit (Hodges & Howieson, 2017), but it allows for assessment and evaluation of the group's (or a team's) learning and implementation experiences. For example, in our evaluation plan, the coaches assess and report on the group's successes and challenges in implementing new skills, practices, and strategies within their programs, organizations, and communities. Further, as researchers/evaluators, we are now early in the process of conducting focus groups with the groups to assess their perceptions, learning and coaching experiences, and outcomes and results of leadership development as individuals and a collective. Some examples of the questions include: *What did you find most valuable or useful about the leadership learning? Can you describe the ways you have been able to apply the knowledge or skills you gained in your work? What is different now than before? Have you trained other people in the ideas or skills you learned, or used any exercises from the learning modules with your staff or in meetings? How effective was the coach's listening, advice, direction, facilitation, and empowerment? How did the coach use opportunities for you to practice implementation of the targeted skills? What were the results of coaching, and specify how beneficial were these results to you, your team/staff, and the organization? As a result of your learning and development, how have you helped your organization to succeed? Overall, what impact have you observed on your effectiveness as an organization/group as a result of training?*

Organizational (program and/or team) performance assessment

Assessing the impact of leadership training on organizational or sector performance has historically been the most difficult aspect of leadership development evaluation – *How beneficial and impactful were the results of an individual's or a group's leadership development to their organization/sector?* Effectively documenting performance improvement in programmatic and/or consumer outcomes as results of leadership development can take various forms. Besides participants' self-reports, we are considering how supervisors and managers in the organization can be surveyed or interviewed to report on and corroborate participants' transfer of learning to assess more effectively and objectively the impact of individual leadership growth on organizational capacity and performance – as demonstrated through changes in work behaviors, performance, and growth mindset (Coloma et al., 2012; Roberts, 2015). *Beyond perceptions, we must ask what team or program performance measures could be examined for those programs or teams whose leaders participated in leadership development activities?* Simply documenting any systems or processes put in place within the organization to align with and help sustain the changed behaviors and results – such as rooting them in performance management, informal and formal feedback reviews or conversations, rewards, mentoring, and redesigning work structures – could be a first step toward assessing the impact of training on organizational capacity and performance.

Tracking performance metrics and measuring progress that is linked to changes in leadership skills and behaviors is more challenging, but also possible. For example, in the large human service agency that is sponsoring all of their managers to participate in the leadership certificate program, we are negotiating with their quality assurance director to compare actual programmatic and/or team performance data at different time points – before leadership development ensued, several months after completion of leadership learning and coaching, and again at a later time to determine what changed in the organization, and in what ways, and how it was influenced by, or a result of, participants' leadership behavior.

Participants, themselves, can build on and extend the benefits of leadership development through the practice of "self-coaching" via continuous reflection, asking the right questions, taking risks, and stretching their newfound competencies (Lobell, Sikka, & Menon, 2017). Journaling their reflections on leadership issues, and documenting implementation successes and challenges, and behaviors or actions that benefit or transform the organization and/or service provision is another mechanism for leadership development evaluation and tracking results. We are exploring this option with the assistance of the coaches within both their peer coaching circles and individual executive coaching with those managers/executive directors who are pursuing additional coaching.

Throughout our commentary, we have highlighted multiple evaluative questions, replicable strategies, and ideas to develop more robust research to better understand and document successful leadership development behaviors, changes in performance, and impact at the individual, collective group/team, and organizational levels (summarized in Figure 1). Ultimately, a goal of leadership development research is to identify which components of a leadership development program may have the greatest outcomes and impact over time. However, realistically, it may prove difficult to isolate the effects of either any specific component of or the leadership development program as a whole from other personal, organizational, and environmental factors, which could affect both individual and organizational outcomes and results. While perpetually challenging, the human service organization and management field is ripe for critical assessment of leadership development expectations, interventions, and investments, and innovation and experimentation with a variety of evaluation strategies to assess leadership training impact at multiple levels.

Disclosure statement

No potential conflict of interest was reported by the authors.

References

Ardichvilli, A., Natt och Dag, K., & Manderscheid, S. (2016). Leadership development: Current and emerging models and practices. *Advances in Developing Human Resources*, 18(3), 275–285. doi:10.1177/1523422316645506

Austin, M. J. (2018). Social work management practice (1917–2017): A history to inform the future. *Social Service Review*, 92(4), 548–616. doi:10.1086/701278

Austin, M. J., Regan, K., Samples, M., Schwartz, S., & Carnochan, S. (2011). Building managerial and organizational capacity in non-profit human service organizations through a leadership development program. *Administration in Social Work*, 35, 258–281. doi:10.1080/03643107.2011.575339

Baker, M. (2014). *Peer-to-peer leadership*. San Francisco, CA: Berrett-Koehler Publishers, Inc.

Beattie, R., Kim, S., Hagen, M., Egan, T., Ellinger, A., & Hamlin, R. (2014). Managerial coaching: A review of the empirical literature and development of a model to guide future practice. *Advances in Developing Human Resources*, 16(2), 184–201. doi:10.1177/1523422313520476

Bernotavicz, F., McDaniel, N., Brittain, C., & Dickinson, N. (2013). Leadership in a changing environment: A leadership model for child welfare. *Administration in Social Work*, 37, 401–417. doi:10.1080/03643107.2012.724362

Coloma, J., Gibson, C., & Packard, T. (2012). Participant outcomes of a leadership development initiative in eight human service organizations. *Administration in Social Work*, 36(4), 4–22. doi:10.1080/03643107.2011.614540

Edwards, G., & Turnbull, S. (2013). Special issue on new paradigms in evaluating leadership development. *Advances in Developing Human Resources, 15*(1), 3–9. doi:10.1177/1523422312467147

Feser, C., Nielsen, N., & Rennie, M. (2017, August). What's missing in leadership development? *McKinsey Quarterly,* pp. 1–5.

Fisher, T., Dietz, J., & Antonakis, J. (2016). Leadership process models: A review and synthesis. *Journal of Management, 43*(6), 1726–1753. doi:10.1177/0149206316682830

Gino, F. (2018, -October). The business case for curiosity. *Harvard Business Review,* pp. 48–57.

Hamman, M., & Spayd, M. (2015). *The agile leader* (pp. 1–16). Redmond, WA: Agile Coaching Institute.

Hanson, B. (2013). The leadership development interface: Aligning leaders and organizations toward more effective leadership learning. *Advances in Developing Human Resources, 15*(1), 106–120. doi:10.1177/1523422312465853

Hassell, B. (2016, March). The problem with executive education. *Chief Learning Officer,* pp. 33–38.

Hodges, J., & Howieson, B. (2017). The challenges of leadership in the third sector. *European Management Journal, 35,* 69–77. doi:10.1016/j.emj.2016.12.006

Hopkins, K., Meyer, M., Cohen-Callow, A., Mattocks, N., & Afkinich, J. (2019). Implementation and impact of results-based accountability learning: Successes and challenges with human service professionals of color in urban agencies. *Race and Justice, 9*(1), 80–94. doi:10.1177/2153368718809835

Hopkins, K., Meyer, M., Shera, W., & Peters, S. (2014). Leadership challenges facing nonprofit human service organizations in a post-recession era. *Human Service Organizations: Management, Leadership, and Governance, 38*(5), 419–422.

The Jensen Group. (2014). *The future of work: Making the future work 2015-2020* (pp. 1–36). New York, NY: Search For a Simpler Way Study.

Kennedy, F., Carroll, B., & Francoeur, J. (2013). Mindset not skill set: Evaluating in new paradigms of leadership development. *Advances in Developing Human Resources, 15*(1), 10–26. doi:10.1177/1523422312466835

Liedtka, J. (2018, September-October). Why design thinking works. *Harvard Business Review,* pp. 72–79.

Lobell, J., Sikka, M., & Menon, P. (2017, March). Self-coaching strategies for nonprofit leaders. *Nonprofit Quarterly,* pp. 1–7.

Meyer, M., & Hopkins, K. (2019). *Follow-up implementation of recommendations.* Report to Joseph and Harvey Meyerhoff Family Charitable Funds. University of Maryland School of Social Work, June 1, 2018 – May 30, 2019.

Moldoveanu, M., & Narayandas, D. (2019, March-April). The future of leadership development. *Harvard Business Review,* pp. 40–48.

Palmer, K., & Blake, D. (2018, November). How to help your employees learn from each other. *Harvard Business Review,* pp. 1–6.

Roberts, J. (2015). *Leading through developing talent.* Columbia, Maryland: Philomathia.

Rofuth, T., & Piepenbring, J. (2020). *Management and leadership in social work.* NY: Springer Publishing, LLC.

Shera, W., & Bejan, R. (2017). A post-masters advanced diploma and a MSW specialization in social service administration: Design, delivery, and assessmentof outcomes. *Human Service Organizations: Management, Leadership, and Governance, 41*(3), 240–251.

Vito, R. (2018). Leadership development in human services: Variations in agency training, organizational investment, participant satisfaction, and succession planning. *Human Service Organization: Management, Leadership, and Governance, 42*(3), 251–266.

Whitney, K. (2016, March). Executive education roadmap. *Chief Learning Officer,* pp. 29–32.

Human Service Organization-Environment Relationships in Relation to Environmental Justice: Old and New Approaches to Macro Practice and Research

Bowen McBeath, Qing Tian, Bin Xu, and Jenifer Huang McBeath

ABSTRACT
The topic of organization-environment relations informs how organizational managers, community leaders, and policymakers and advocates secure essential resources, justify their strategic importance, collaborate and compete, and engage in civic participation and politics. Yet the topic has rarely focused upon the built and natural environments; and research on environmental justice (as a sister of social justice) has lagged despite longstanding concerns of environmental racism and strong interest in the development and sustainment of community-based practices, programs, and policies in response to environmental degradation. We provide a brief vision of macro practice, education, research, and theory that is (1) centered in environmental justice and (2) rooted in what managers and leaders do within organizations and communities. Our analysis identifies novel and needed directions for the future, as we imply that important theoretical and conceptual perspectives supporting macro practice, programming, and research are being unmoored by environmental dislocations facing targeted communities.

Organization-environment relationships is a core topic of this journal, concerning how human service organizations and management ("HSO&M") secure essential resources, justify their strategic importance, collaborate and compete with formal organizations and informal associations, and advocate and engage politically. Yet research on HSO&M has rarely focused upon the built and natural environments, environmental disaster management, or immigrant and refugee management (for exceptions, see Kim and Zakour (2018) and Smith (2012)). Critically, attention to environmental justice (as a sister of social justice) is mostly absent from the journal.

Organizational, managerial, and community environmental needs are expected to rise in the future due to environmental dislocation resulting from the movement of industry and capital goods as well as from extreme weather events. Industrial and natural disasters are high-impact events that disproportionately affect communities of color; and the UN Intergovernmental Panel on Climate Change (Intergovernmental Panel on Climate Change, 2018) and US National Climate Assessment (US Global Change Research Program, 2018) suggest that such events can be expected to worsen due to climate

A previous version of this commentary was presented at the January 2019 Society for Social Work and Research Pre-Conference Meeting on "The Future of Human Service Organizational and Management Research". We express our deep appreciation to the anonymous peer reviewers, whose excellent suggestions helped to improve the paper. Support from the National Natural Science Foundation of China for the research project "Research on Human Perception and Adaptation Behavior to Climate Change by Tracking Study: Making Northeast China as a Case (No. 41471155)" is gratefully acknowledged. The perspectives expressed and errors and omissions are ours.

change (Xu, Ramanathan, & Victor, 2018). In alignment with proposals envisioning public policy and community development strategies to address extreme weather and climate change (Mason & Rigg, 2019), human service organizations are often formally charged with responding to immediate demands for environmentally-focused emergency services, coordination with critical systems (i.e., healthcare, housing, education, and food/water safety), and ongoing programming and delivery of public services and goods (Kapucu & Kuotsai, 2014). Yet we question whether HSO&M advocates, researchers, and scholars are doing enough to support environmental issues.

The specific aim of our commentary is to provide a brief vision of HSO&M practice, research, and theory that is centered in environmental justice, as agency and community leaders and social work practitioners are challenged to respond to environmental dilemmas facing contested intersectionalities – i.e., poor peoples and communities of color coping with the detritus of industrialization and deindustrialization in minoritized geographies. More generally for HSO&M researchers and theorists, our purpose is to push for more attention to the complex social ecology of the built and natural environments as an essential aspect of organization-environment relationships. The approach to research and theory is rooted in macro practice, with its intersecting domains of community, organizational and management, and policy practice – in particular in the efforts of community-based organizations and the strategic activities of leaders and other key stakeholders.

Our commentary is premised upon a theoretical perspective that frames the intersections among HSO&M and the environment within a complex institutional context. Normatively, we suggest that human service organizations play a mediating institutional role in connecting policies, programs, and frontline practice (Collins-Camargo, Chuang, & McBeath, 2019; Mosley, 2014), thereby supporting human service populations and other groups at great risk of experiencing major environmental dilemmas. In addressing environmental needs in low-income, diverse community contexts, HSO&M should occupy an informal, important position in connecting environmental advocacy to policy-making through civic participation and community development. Others have carefully described the contested terrain occupied by advocates and organizers working in partnership with and/or in opposition to HSO&M and other community-based organizations (Doering-White, 2018; Mathias, 2018); our commentary touches only lightly upon these complexities.

Our concern is more basic, centered in a premise that organizational and managerial capacity is needed for community stakeholders to actively compete for representation in diverse civic and policy spheres (Despard, Ansong, Nafziger-Mayegun, & Adjabeng, 2018; Kearns, 2006). From a social and environmental justice perspective, policy and program experimentation should be evaluated in relation to the needs of those populations and communities most affected by and least able to adapt to environmental dislocation. Community needs assessment should be accompanied by HSO&M needs assessments relating to fiscal, infrastructural, managerial, and frontline service capacity to respond to environmental dilemmas. Yet capacity building and sustainment (focusing upon the provision of interorganizational, organizational, and administrative supports over time) is underdeveloped among HSO&M practitioners and environmental advocates; and is understudied among HSO&M researchers, particularly from interpretivist and critical perspectives.

Our commentary provides examples of current policies and practices drawn principally from the Grand Challenges for Social Work, and we highlight practice- and theory-informed research to be developed. Yet we also touch upon some underpinnings of classic organization-environment frameworks in order to advocate for greater attention to their connective tissues (i.e., to unpack key assumptions and central premises). As a result, our commentary straddles two levels: (1) we call for more attention to environmental justice among HSO&M practitioners and researchers; and (2) we imply that important theoretical and conceptual perspectives supporting HSO&M practice, programming, and research may become unmoored by future dislocations facing targeted communities (e.g., "climate apartheid" (UNHRC, 2019)).

These two levels are not mutually distinct. Instead and as summarized in Table 1, they cohere around a belief that future opportunities for macro practice, education, research, and theorizing are needed to connect HSO&M and environmental justice. Some of these opportunities reflect the perspectives of less-familiar disciplines, organizations, and communities. However, some of what we

Table 1. Connecting HSO&M and environmental justice: directions for future macro practice, education, research, and theory.

Practice

(1) Within human service organizations at the executive and board governance levels, review and update agency disaster preparedness plans and track progress toward environmental equity.

(2) Ensure that sufficient interorganizational, organizational, and managerial capacity exists to address community environmental needs. If such capacity does not exist, then advocate for additional supports with public agencies and foundations.

(3) Expand environmental justice-focused service coproduction and co-leadership initiatives, particularly to support community development for poor peoples and communities of color.

(4) Incentivize collaborative networks of human service organizations and environmental services, disaster planning and response, and community development organizations in order to develop coordinated, flexible, and targeted responses to community environmental problems.

(5) Turn knowledge sharing of successful community environmental practices and programs into political advocacy and policy involvement.

Education

(6) Draw upon faculty expertise and leadership to integrate environmental justice and the built and natural environments into social work courses on practice, field education, human behavior and the social environment, policy, research, and diversity, equity, and inclusion.

(7) Focusing specifically on the social work macro practice courses of community practice, HSO&M practice, and policy practice, balance the historic emphasis on problem-oriented practice with attention to solution-oriented environmental justice strategies that involve interorganizational collaboration, local leadership, service coproduction, and community health promotion and healing.

(8) Support a university-wide commitment to environmental justice by identifying common degree programs, cross-listing relevant courses across disciplines and professional schools, providing seed grants for faculty and students to initiate pilot demonstrations, and developing public lectures on related topics (e.g., strategies to address the Grand Challenge of climate change).

(9) Build university-industry innovation hubs to promote local and regional practice, program, and policy responses to environmental degradation.

(10) Connect leading higher education associations (e.g., Council on Social Work Education, National Association of Social Workers, Society for Social Work and Research) in order to share curricular, practice, and research approaches to environmental justice.

Research

(11) Root research on HSO&M more actively within the community environmental and socioeconomic context.

(12) Study how leaders within human service organizations are responding to environmental racism and supporting environmental health in minoritized communities.

(13) Evaluate the impacts of environmental policies and programs on communities, and examine how human service organizations are adapting to and/or mitigating environmental policy/program effects.

(14) Orient HSO&M research approaches around community-based, participatory, and service user-centered epistemologies, with a goal of using research to reduce environmental injustice and enhance community participation and resilience.

(15) Methodologically, supplement the common use of organizational surveys and brief interviews of senior managers and leaders ("broad and narrow evidence") with cultural knowledge as well as narrative methods of inquiry (e.g., storytelling) to support deeper investigation of processes of organizational and community change in response to environmental dilemmas.

Theory

(16) Incorporate theoretical attention to environmental justice in relation to other PESTLE domains (i.e., factors pertaining to politics, economics, sociocultural determinants, technology, laws, and the environment).

(17) Anticipate the need to use non-traditional organizational theories to explain HSO&M responses to exogenous institutional shocks such as extreme weather and disasters.

(18) Center macro practice theorizing – theory development, refinement/adaptation, and use – within local/indigenous perspectives and in collaboration with organizational leaders.

(19) Unpack the key metaphors driving macro practice, policy, and research (e.g., environmental management vs. environmental stewardship vs. environmental transformation).

(20) Craft new theories across scope and scale, to account for different understandings of intensity, timeframe, and geography (ranging from "quick-and-dirty", episodic, and smaller-scale processes of change to longer-term, slower, more sustained, and larger-scale processes of change).

"HSO&M" = human service organizational and management.

are arguing for is familiar but may get neglected, particularly as macro practitioners and researchers are increasingly cloistering ourselves into the specialized fields of community practice, HSO&M practice, and policy practice. As embodied in our subtitle, our commentary therefore contains an argument for old and new approaches to macro practice and research.

We organize our commentary via three sections. We first set the stage by briefly synthesizing and reflecting upon what is known concerning our topic. In the second section, we identify three tensions in environmental practice within and between human service organizations. The concluding section reflects briefly upon these specific issues in order to identify broader implications for future macro practice, education, research, and theory.

Situating HSO&M in relation to environmental justice

Current practice conceptualizations

Environmental justice has been described as "the marriage of the movement for social justice with environmentalism" (McGurty, 1997, p. 303, quoted in Philip & Reisch, 2015) that "highlights the linkage between environmental degradation and power imbalances as the mainly human victims of environmental degradation also must contend with injustices related to class, gender, race, ethnicity, and locale" (Powers, Willett, Mathias, & Hayward, 2018, p. 74). As an action concept, environmental justice involves efforts to address environmental disasters as well as slower-moving environmental dilemmas (notably industrialization and deindustrialization) disproportionately affecting low-income, minoritized communities due to inequitable power and resources (Dominelli, 2013). It is understood to foster empowerment through knowledge and behavior at multiple levels of practice, including at: individual and group levels; organizational and community levels; and the societal level (particularly in regards to the policy/governance efforts of social and political institutions in relation to market actors). The overall intention is to redress inequities of public resources and correct imbalances in public decision-making in response to environmental disasters and for environmental health promotion (National Environmental Health Partnership Council, 2016).

From a normative lens reflected in the NASW Code of Ethics, social work professionals and organizations should be expected to address social and environmental justice. A similar emphasis is shared by the Academy of Management. George and colleagues (2014) posit that organizations should: explain socially- and environmentally-sustainable values and support goal attainment; address unjust barriers by resolving organizational constraints; foster coordination and collaboration at different levels of analysis; and enhance societal outcomes and impacts. Promotive strategies at the societal level include: understanding and reshaping supply and value chains; supporting organizational resilience and adaptation; and understanding societal shifts in work and life (Howard-Grenville, Buckle, Hoskins, & George, 2014). At the organizational and interorganizational level, strategies include participatory practice approaches centered in local community experimentation (Ferraro, Etzion, & Gehman, 2015).

Social work scholars have identified the need for environmental social work practice knowledge. Dominelli (2018) states, "Green social work reshapes social work's generic skills by emphasizing the coproduction of knowledge and action in transdisciplinary, empowering processes that operate before a disaster, throughout it and afterward in reconstruction endeavors. It does so by engaging local residents in the development of resilience as people and communities recover from the impact of a disaster" (pp. 13–14). Community change strategies include consciousness raising, advocating, and lobbying; community mobilization; and dialoging with residents, policymakers, and the media (Dominelli, 2018). Practitioner roles include facilitator, coordinator, planner, mobilizer, negotiator, mediator, advocate, educator, researcher, trainer, translator, and therapist (Dominelli, 2013; Philip & Reisch, 2015).

These environmental practice strategies fit comfortably within general macro practice methods, including: facilitating groups; supervision; developing, coordinating, and managing resources;

negotiation and managing conflict and change; leadership; analyzing, planning, and leading on critical community, organizational, and policy issues; program development, implementation, and evaluation; advocacy, lobbying, public education, and developing coalitions; social marketing and public speaking; and using assets-based approaches to facilitate the empowerment of diverse stakeholders (Reisch, 2019). These practice approaches can also be situated in relation to existing HSO&M practice competencies, including those promulgated by the Network for Social Work Management in the areas of executive leadership, resource management, strategic management, and community collaboration.

For instance, a community-based leadership development program might seek to promote community resilience via an initiative to address neighborhood toxic waste. Program aims might include fostering communication and dialog across different levels of practice and among different stakeholders, thereby promoting collaborative knowledge sharing and problem solving. At the program level, management staff might secure resources to partner with community leaders around residents' environmental education and civic participation efforts. At the organizational level, the initiative might be: housed within a culturally specific multiservice nonprofit human service organization; funded by public grants and contracts (e.g., city, county, state, and/or regional consortia) and private philanthropic donations; and administered by a nonprofit board and director who are accountable for program management and organizational governance. At the community level, nonprofit human service directors might develop strategic alliances with service, educational, and advocacy organizations to promote environmentally-focused policy and program changes. Organizational leaders might therefore be expected to support HSO&M competency development to respond to current environmental dilemmas.

Current theoretical, research, and educational approaches and knowledge gaps

From an institutional theoretical perspective, evidence of new organizational roles and practice linkages involving HSO&M and the environment reflect: strategic emphasis upon the "triple bottom line" of social, economic, and environmental sustainability in organizational and interorganizational initiatives (Chi, Chong, Ng, & Busiol, 2019; Mor Barak, In press); and MSW and non-MSW electives and required courses dedicated to ecosocial practice and green social work (Beltran, Hacker, & Begun, 2016; Cuadra & Eydal, 2018; Nipperess & Boddy, 2018). However, research on social work management, public and nonprofit management, and business management – in which one would expect to find scholarship pertaining to HSO&M – generally has not incorporated environmental issues, and has largely shied away from environmental justice.

For example, in this journal the topic of human service organization-environment dynamics commonly concerns collaborative and competitive relationships involving diverse funders, normative bodies (educational institutions, accrediting bodies), providers, and service users, with research distinguishing between within-organizational vs. extra-organizational factors in response to external challenges (Gummer, 1997; Mulroy, 2004; Schmid, 2004; Watson & Hegar, 2013). Although analysis of intra- and inter-organizational relationships can involve research on PESTLE domains (i.e., factors pertaining to politics, economics, sociocultural determinants, technology, laws, and the environment), little research and curricular attention is generally dedicated to the latter. Moreover, such analysis can be used to enhance competitive advantage in terms of market share, profits, and "business as usual" (Wright & Nyberg, 2017). Finally, while a literature in business and public/nonprofit management concerns social sustainability (Moldavanova & Goerdel, 2018), attention to environmental sustainability is arguably more the exception than the norm.

Conversely, literatures on the topics of environmental justice and environmental sustainability have traditionally concerned events affecting human health and environmental wellbeing. In the environmental sciences and the professions of urban planning and natural resource management, a substantial literature identifies the web of political and social institutions and complex organizations – often termed "social-ecological systems" (Orach & Schlüter, 2016) – involved in mitigating/adapting to anthropogenic hazards. We reflect briefly upon this literature in our next section. Additionally, public health efforts identify the need for and testing/improvement of community-based environmental health interventions (National Environmental Health Partnership Council, 2016).

Finally, a small, robust literature situates social work macro practice in relation to the environment. Social work research and education have focused upon the involvement of advocates and organizers in organizational settings ranging from informal community associations to international NGOs in response to natural and industrial disasters as well as environmental violence/racism (e.g., urban brownfields in communities of color, fracking and waste disposal in rural communities, water/land sovereignty challenges in indigenous and tribal communities). (Reviews of this literature include: Krings, Victor, Mathias, & Perron, In press; Mason, Shires, Arwood, & Borst, 2017; Ramsay & Boddy, 2017).

Yet overall, the conceptual cupboard is not as full as one might like to see. Too little HSO&M theory and research examines environmental justice initiatives': organizational remit, efforts, and spheres of influence vis-à-vis other community-based providers and institutions; practice methods and workforce involvement; opportunities for collaboration and/or competition; and consequences for community stakeholders, organizations, and institutionalized systems. In addition, we are aware of very few macro social work educational initiatives – and none that is specific to HSO&M – that focus upon the environment. As aforementioned, Table 1 identifies directions for macro practice education, research, and theory.

Tensions in environmental practice within and between human service organizations

The Grand Challenges for Social Work ("GCSW") to "Create Social Responses to a Changing Environment" (Kemp & Palinkas, 2015) provides the clearest prescription to date regarding how policymakers and practitioners should respond to environmental risks. It envisions a mature, multi-stage approach to environmental disaster response resulting from extreme weather events. The specific GCSW is organized around the interrelated subjects of: disaster preparedness/response involving prevention and mitigation; refugee resettlement and integration to address population dislocation; community-level capacity building, organizing, and development to promote adaptation, resilience, and sustainability; and policy, community-based advocacy, and public education to mitigate/target the causes of environmental change.

Concerning the subject of pre-disaster preparedness, during-disaster services, and post-disaster response, the focus includes: Tier 1 interventions to address ecosocial impacts related to health, cleanup, economic redevelopment, and employment/training; Tier 2 interventions, in which community leadership is needed to facilitate social supports and risk reduction; and Tier 3 interventions involving the use of individual and family EBPs to reduce psychosocial impacts and foster resilience. These interventions involve connections with disaster response, human service, healthcare, educational, and agricultural systems; and are comparable in many respects to other national policy statements (e.g., National Environmental Health Partnership Council, 2016).

We use the specific GCSW as an example to draw attention to three implementation issues pertaining to how HSO&M adapt to environmental dilemmas. The first concerns the need for organizational and management supports to make environmental policies, programs, and practices work better. The second concerns the contested spaces that arise whenever participatory environmental initiatives are enacted within human service organizations. And the third concerns the theoretical and practical question of transformation and sustainability of environmental policy and practice interventions. Each of these three issues distinguishes between environmental disaster management (the province of HSO&M practice) vs. the messy movement toward environmental justice (the province of community and policy practice).

Essential organizational and managerial supports can be hard to secure

First, organizational development and management support are needed to ensure that environmental policies and practices are not done "to and for" poor peoples and communities of color. In relation to the specific GCSW, research alludes to the importance of organizations and management as leaders are tasked with facilitating disaster response and promoting community environmental resilience. Human service executives can struggle post-disaster with: significant and changing service needs of community residents; physical infrastructural damage; fiscal concerns (notably insufficient cash flow and reserves); administrative coverage gaps and staffing needs, including personnel losses; and intra- and interorganizational communication and collaboration challenges (Chikoto-Schultz, 2016; Simo & Bies, 2007; Smith, 2012). Other evidence suggests that environmental justice advocates can have significant organizational development needs in the areas of: resource development and operations management; media, campaign, and strategic planning; lobbying and national/local politics; and interorganizational and community-focused coalition building (Cwikel & Blit-Cohen, 2018; Kapucu & Kuotsai, 2014; Maglaglic, 2019).

Thus, a key outgrowth of the literature on organization-environment relations is that the implementation of community-based policy and program initiatives requires sufficient capacity at the managerial, organizational, and interorganizational levels – i.e., collaborative knowledge, technical expertise, funding, leadership, teamwork, prosocial norms, cultural strengths, and training and assistance (Droppa & Giunta, 2015; Schmid, 2019). This thesis also holds for perspectives on the implementation and diffusion of EBPs, evidence-informed practice, and evidence-based management involving multiple agencies and systems of care (Damschroder et al., 2009; Rousseau & Gunia, 2016; Willging, Gunderson, Green, Jaramillo, & Garrison et al., 2018).

We worry that new environmental initiatives will be started and sustained by larger, better prepared HSO&M (i.e., those with sufficiently experienced and robust organizational supports and interorganizational partnerships). We are also concerned that in a climate of scarcity, competition for resources among larger organizations (to fund ongoing and new initiatives) may crowd out smaller, fledgling efforts. These latter organizations and associations are likely to reflect communities of color and local, evolving service needs. For example, in summarizing results from small to medium nonprofit culturally-based providers over a three-year period in the wake of Hurricane Katrina, Smith (2012) concluded, "After a catastrophe, organizations try to work together. As short-term funding goes away and private contractors emerge, competition returns" (p. 377).

Finally, at a practical and theoretical level, we are concerned that in a market-oriented political economy, agency dependence upon and competition for grants and contracts to secure community-based emergency services and ongoing community assistance may contribute to the emergence of a collective action problem – where organizations make individually sensible decisions that result in collectively dysfunctional outcomes. Such negative outcomes may include the loss of culturally specific services, decreased equity and inclusion, poorer environmental health, and insufficient preparation for future adverse disasters.

Illuminating tensions in human service coproduction in relation to environmental justice

Second, our interest in the specific GCSW relates to how human service organizations can codevelop and coproduce in supporting environmental justice and other community-based initiatives. In coproduced services, public service delivery involves some essential level of "citizen" knowledge and involvement in service planning and delivery (using the original concept by Elinor Ostrom, which evolved to "customer" in the New Public Management era, followed more recently by "service user") (Brandsen, Steen, & Vershuere, 2018). As described earlier, an environmentally just approach to the "slow violence" (Willett, 2019) that minoritized communities experience might be framed around community engagement via diverse ways of knowing (particularly indigenous and cultural knowledge), mobilization, and community healing (Ginwright, 2015). Interorganizationally, local leaders might serve as: brokers, in connecting needed external funding with new and ongoing programming; and gatekeepers, in protecting community members who fear reprisal from dominant institutions (Alston, 2019; Teixeira & Krings, 2015). Within organizations, efforts could involve co-leadership roles of service users and organizational representatives in environmental education, planning, development, service delivery, and improvement.

Yet coproduction is a variable, not a constant. Targeted communities should be rightly apprehensive that their roles may be tokenized, that their opportunities for self-determination may be limited, and that too few opportunities may exist for local leadership and community development. Therefore, essential questions concern the conditions under which human services are more environmentally just, and how human service organizations, managers, and frontline practitioners can partner in coproducing services.

Reflecting a critical institutionalist approach, human service organizations can serve as sites of contestation, conflict, and compromise within as well as across organizations and other formal bodies (Eriksson & Bjerge, 2019; Lok, 2019; Thornton, Ocasio, & Lounsbury, 2012). Managers and community stakeholders within complex organizations may bring diverse interests and perspectives to a particular environmental issue. They can acquiesce, ignore, reject, buffer, adapt, and innovate in response to internal and external forces (e.g., policy, funding, and market pressures) (Cleaver & De Koning, 2015). Service users, workers, and managers can as a result bring influence internally and externally. Internally, they can shape and be informed (or not) by diverse organizational values, norms, structures, and processes to be more environmentally involved. Externally, agents can individually and collectively shape (or not) diverse environmental interests and perspectives into advocacy (Wang, Liu, & Dang, 2018).

Underlying these possibilities is a more nuanced perspective on the boundedly rational actor approach to HSO&M, in which organizations are structured by managers seeking to improve goal attainment amidst ambiguity, uncertainty, and tradeoffs (i.e., managers as airplane captains). In contrast, critical perspectives – e.g., that identify managers as wielders of instruments of domination/oppression, and/or managers as facilitators, partners, allies, or even accomplices – pose questions as to how directors and staff intersect with power, privilege, and funding to promote agency at the individual, group, and community levels. These questions strike at the heart of organization-environment relations, and are not simple theoretical exercises as they relate to the practical realities of supporting service users in complex organizations (Austin, 2018). In sum, practice-informed theory building and research on environmental justice-focused service user coproduction is most needed to support macro practice curriculum development and sharing of lessons learned with executives and community leaders.

How transformative and sustainable can environmental justice interventions be? How transformative and sustainable are our existing human service interventions?

Third, running through the literature on environmental justice is the question of transformation and sustainability of social-ecological systems and human services. An aphorism on the management of organizational change is that in order for leaders to turn small wins into major accomplishments, their organizations also need to be supported and successful (Stouten, Rousseau, & De Cremer, 2018). For example, in asking how a community-based initiative can be more anti-oppressive and transformative, one can first examine how human service organizations can be more: service user-centered and focused upon community healing; participatory and less hierarchical; culturally humble; and collectivist and liberatory (Chow & Austin, 2008; Ginwright, 2015; McBeath, 2015; Ramsundarsingh & Shier, 2019).

A concern with this question is that dominant HSO&M frameworks can be quite bureaucratic – reflecting industrial and post-industrial (service sector) practice approaches. Core organization-environment theories have been situated within traditional socio-technical methods of management practice and education (e.g., strategic planning and logic modeling, frontline service delivery in alignment with program promising practices and EBPs, performance management and continuous quality improvement).

Perspectives have also included classic and new institutional and political economic approaches involving managerial and organizational adaptation (to formal rules and policies and informal norms) as well as interorganizational competition and collaboration. Some critiques of these theories have identified an overwhelming emphasis upon similarity, persistence, and control at the managerial, organizational, and institutional level (Robinson, 2007). More recently, critical commentaries have noted concerns with neoliberal organizational retrenchment and managerialism driven by a focus upon ensuring public (and private) funding based upon elite governmental priorities (Harlow, Berg, Barry, & Chandler, 2013; Hasenfeld & Garrow, 2012; Yan, Cheung, Tsui, & Chu, 2017). Such concerns might imply that transformative change is unlikely, even in human service organizations that market themselves to be community-based.

Yet we suspect that different HSO&M theoretical lenses will support very different research studies and may shape their eventual findings. From a meso-organizational perspective, strategic management theory may suggest that HSO&M leaders can envision different ways to develop new environmental initiatives, including: in-house development of new social enterprises; subcontracting with a separate environmental justice provider to supply needed expertise; and strategic alliance formation involving two or more organizations to develop complementary service programs, enhance resources and technical knowledge, and collaborate to provide new services to existing community members and/or existing services to new community members (Shier & Handy, 2015). These possibilities can range from less risky to riskier (economically, socially, and politically) in terms of the alignment of organizations': core values and goals; knowledge and service technology; funding relationships; accountability systems; and market dynamics, including community memberships.

From a macro-organizational perspective, the adaptive governance literature provides examples of how networks of institutions and organizations coordinate in response to environmental dilemmas, and engage in organizational learning and shared problem-solving amidst ambiguity and complexity. (Reviews of the literature include: Berkes, 2009; Karpouzoglou, Dewulf, & Clark, 2016; Sharma-Wallace, Velarde, & Wreford, 2018). Some of these initiatives have involved non-traditional funders and actors, and overall have varied by: purpose (transactive, adaptive, transformative); sector (public, nonprofit, for-profit); legal-jurisdictional involvement (local, regional, state, national, supra-national); nature of change over time (short-term vs. long-term, episodic vs. consistent, incremental vs. punctuated equilibrium); and governance mechanism (formal tools such as charters/constitutions, rules, policies, and contracts, as well as informal norms such as trust and reciprocity). If there has been a basic tenor to the initiatives, it is that they have had strong institutional sponsors and network leaders – notably progressive political leaders and expert public administrators supported by local/regional governmental councils (Chong, Chi, & Busiol, 2019) – and they have tended to reject "either/or" approaches in favor of "both/and" approaches to institutional design.

The following theoretical prompts may help to identify "both/and" possibilities for meso- and macro-organizational research involving HSO&M and environmental justice.

- Anticipating the need to address common-pool resource issues across distinct geographies. For example, how can community leaders (including HSO&M) in communities/states/nations bounded by major rivers ensure continued access to water and arable land for human consumption and agricultural-industrial production?
- Moving from an oversimplified problem-oriented practice approach, to a wicked problem situation (in which organizational and community problems and solutions may be messy), and then to a policy streams perspective (involving problems, policy options, politics, and organizational entrepreneurs (Vangen, Hayes, & Cornforth, 2015). For example, in a VUCA world (i.e., volatile, uncertain, complex, ambiguous), how do human service executives respond to local floods/fires, and prioritize community-based solutions? What workable strategies prevent organizational myopia and management-by-"burying head in the sand"?
- Conceptualizing the involvement of HSO&M as "first responders" for community environmental development. First responder organizations generally involve disaster response and emergency services; secondary responders provide support to first responders; and tertiary responders rebuild

basic infrastructure and provide needed healthcare and community services. However, in a community development context focused upon resiliency, how can HSO&M envision "first responder" roles in environmental justice programs and environmental education initiatives, particularly if a scenario of climate apartheid (UNHRC, 2019) becomes a reality?

In sum, while some well-known HSO&M-environment frameworks are well-theorized, others should be explored – particularly those that support theorizing of local problem-solving in response to longstanding environmental dilemmas. For example, we are reminded that in response to severe droughts over decades in northern China, governmental agricultural water management projects have at great cost supported and monitored local infrastructure for ancient irrigation canals (Dalin, Hanasaki, Qiu, Mauzerall, & Rodriguez-Iturbe, 2014). These canals have existed for hundreds of years, and have helped to bring water from rivers to rural communities. We are therefore interested in theory-informed research on how local institutions and community-based organizations, including HSO&M, address extreme climatic events resulting in slower-moving, longer-term impacts spread over larger spatio-temporal scales. And we suspect that narrative-based and historical studies will support small-scale theory building regarding how institutions and organizations can sustain environmental resilience (Moezzi, Janda, & Rotmann, 2017).

Regardless of the particular theory in use, we believe that research on transformation and sustainability should be attentive to the core outcomes reflected in Figure 1. Research is needed to help managers anticipate and respond to place- and race-based environmental challenges – starting with reviews of disaster preparedness plans, in tandem with individual/group and organizational inventories and gap analysis. At the community level, studies of environmental justice programs involving community-based organizations are essential. Moreover, policy research should evaluate: how community residents are responding to major environmental changes (including extreme weather and climate); and whether specific environmental and social welfare policies and governance are reducing social and environmental inequities (Alston, 2019; Mason & Rigg, 2019). One should not have to choose between good theory and good evidence. But given the lack of relevant HSO&M studies to date, we would argue for more of the latter in order to support environmental advocacy and the crafting of new, vibrant theories.

Individual and Group Level

Residents' experiences, including their knowledge, attitudes, behaviors (including opposition), needs, reactions, and concerns in relation to environmental challenges. Understanding of their experiences should reflect emic and etic lenses.

Organizational Level

Delivery of needed services (e.g., accessibility, sufficiency, quality, effectiveness, equity) in response to disasters and other environmental dilemmas; funding, leadership, teamwork, and other essential capacities of managers and organizations to support service coproduction; intraorganizational and interorganizational coordination and collaboration; and involvement in politics and advocacy.

Community Level

Social-environmental civic capacity, trauma reduction, culturally centered healing, resilience, and health and wellbeing.

Policy-Institutional Level

The involvement of HSO&M in relation to markets and social welfare and environmental policy spheres (to map the complex interorganizational ecology of disaster management); and the implementation and governance of human services and related systems in response to environmental dilemmas. Attention should be paid to inter-professional and cross-jurisdictional collaboration and competition.

Figure 1. Key environmental justice outcomes by level of analysis.

Toward the future

We now draw connections between our discussion of the specific topic (regarding HSO&M practice and environmental justice) and the future of macro research, education, and theory. First, we strongly encourage the American Academy of Social Work and Social Welfare (the coordinating body of the GCSW) to advocate for stronger institutional research pipelines. Specifically, research funding is needed to support macro practice research – particularly community and organizational needs assessments and capacity building studies – in order to reduce community environmental injustice. By definition, Grand Challenges require the development of government-academic-industry networks to transform applied scientific research into practice and program innovations (McBeath et al., 2019). Other scientific societies acknowledge the importance of institutional supports for research-practice partnerships in their Grand Challenges (George, Howard-Grenville, Joshi, & Thanyi, 2014; Reid et al., 2010). These societies also serve as knowledge coordinating bodies, within which leading universities collaborate and compete to advance applied science to address practical problems. We look forward to the development of policy-university-industry hubs to address GCSW "moon shots", including the specific challenge concerning the environment.

Research-to-practice pipelines do not come cheap and are not built overnight. Future development of macro practice educational initiatives focused upon environmental justice will also require substantial investments, but in comparison may present clearer and simpler targets. Practice courses on management and leadership, program development and policy implementation, organizational change, and social entrepreneurship should be able to incorporate an emphasis on environmental justice. Yet a longstanding concern is sufficient numbers of macro practice faculty with the requisite expertise and interest to revise existing curricula and develop new courses and certificate programs. If faculty do not have such expertise in-house (particularly in environmental policymaking and advocacy, environmental management, and disaster management), then external opportunities for curricular and training partnerships should be incentivized.

In envisioning a future focused upon HSO&M-environmental justice research studies, we reaffirm the importance of research on service coproduction via the development, implementation, and sustainment of participatory programs and practices. The intention is to use research to ensure that organizational decision-making, programming, and governance are centered in community resilience and healing, particularly as leaders seek participatory ways to address social-environmental disasters and public health crises. This supports a more expansive vision of community engagement and involvement beyond tokenistic service on boards and advisory committees, and beyond the hiring of occasional community members.

More evidence is needed of participatory, anti-oppressive initiatives, particularly given the organizational maintenance demands of HSO&M to "keep the lights on" (Hasenfeld & Garrow, 2012; McBeath, 2015; Mosley, 2012). On this front, old and new research and theory are needed to connect organizational/management practice and community practice. For example, researchers focused upon environmental justice might explore connections between (a) organizing amidst organization and (b) transformation in relation to adaptation. Organizing to support transformation is traditionally the remit of community practitioners, whereas organization to support adaptation is arguably the province of HSO&M practitioners (Austin, 1986; Gummer, 1997). All four cells of the proverbial 2 × 2 table are needed to examine the coproduction and sustainment of transformative environmental justice initiatives.

Our commentary concludes with a call for a renewed commitment to researching and theorizing organization-environment relations, accompanied by interpretivist and critical perspectives. Many of the basic considerations we shared can be applied to other environmental dilemmas as well as other PESTLE domains. In particular, the suggestions provided in Table 1 and Figure 1 can support studies of how human service organizations respond to external contingencies and dependencies (e.g., research on how HSO&M anticipate and respond to decreased state service contracts and/or EBP requirements due to rapidly changing public policies; studies of HSO&M advocacy in response to community calls for racial equity).

For research and theories to be used and useful, they should be attentive to the practice needs of organizational and community leaders and other key stakeholders charged with responding to environmental and social injustice. Research on the interconnections of HSO&M and the environment should seek to enhance theory development, by teasing apart conceptual ties, exploring underdeveloped concepts and practices, and contesting theories across professions and disciplines. (A similar argument can be made for the other five PESTLE domains).

Yet it is not clear that approaches used by other disciplines and professions can be easily and effectively put into practice in HSO&M and social work. HSO&M research and theory will therefore benefit from sustained examination and cross-pollination with seemingly unrelated professions and disciplines also dedicated to environmental and social justice (e.g., environmental education, urban planning, rural development). In addition, opportunities for international macro practice research and education are likely to present themselves as countries, cultures, and communities explore different methods for promoting environmental justice.

Disclosure statement

No potential conflict of interest was reported by the authors.

References

Alston, M. (2019). Gender, politics, and water in Australia and Bangladesh. In L. R. Mason & J. Rigg (Eds.), *People and climate change: Vulnerability, adaptation, and social justice* (pp. 165–183). New York, NY: Oxford University Press.

Austin, M. J. (1986). Community organization and social administration: Partnership or irrelevance? *Human Service Organizations: Management, Leadership, & Governance, 10*, 27–39.

Austin, M. J. (2018). Social work management practice, 1917-2017: A history to inform the future. *Social Service Review, 92*, 548–616. doi:10.1086/701278

Beltran, R., Hacker, A., & Begun, A. (2016). Environmental justice is a social justice issue: Incorporating environmental justice in social work practice curricula. *Journal of Social Work Education, 52*, 493–502. doi:10.1080/10437797.2016.1215277

Berkes, F. (2009). Evolution of co-management: Role of knowledge generation, bridging organizations and social learning. *Journal of Environmental Management, 90*, 1692–1702. doi:10.1016/j.jenvman.2008.12.001

Brandsen, T., Steen, T., & Vershuere, B. (2018). Co-creation and co-production in public services: Urgent issues in practice and research. In T. Brandsen, T. Steen, & B. Vershuere (Eds.), *Co-creation and co-production: Engaging citizens in public services* (pp. 3–8). New York, NY: Routledge.

Chi, I., Chong, A. M. L., Ng, T. K., & Busiol, D. (2019). Social work and sustainable development: An overview. In A. M. L. Chong & I. Chi (Eds.), *Social work and sustainability in Asia: Facing the challenges of global environmental changes* (pp. 3–20). New York, NY: Routledge.

Chikoto-Schultz, G. L. (2016). Nonprofits and disasters. In D. C. Downey (Ed.), *Cities and disasters* (pp. 27–52). New York, NY: CRC Press.

Chong, A. M. L., Chi, I., & Busiol, D. (2019). Leadership and sustainable development in the future. In A. M. L. Chong & I. Chi (Eds.), *Social work and sustainability in Asia: Facing the challenges of global environmental changes* (pp. 225–251). New York, NY: Routledge.

Chow, J. C. C., & Austin, M. J. (2008). The culturally responsive social service agency: The application of an evolving definition to a case study. *Human Service Organizations: Management, Leadership, & Governance, 32*, 39–64.

Cleaver, F., & De Koning, J. (2015). Furthering critical institutionalism. *International Journal of the Commons, 9*, 1–18. doi:10.18352/ijc.605

Collins-Camargo, C., Chuang, E., & McBeath, B. (2019). Staying afloat amidst the tempest: External pressures facing private child and family serving agencies and strategies employed to address them. *Human Service Organizations: Management, Leadership, & Governance, 43*, 125–145.

Cuadra, C. B., & Eydal, G. B. (2018). Towards a curriculum in disaster risk reduction from a green social work perspective. In L. Dominelli (Ed.), *The Routledge handbook of green social work* (pp. 522–534). New York, NY: Routledge.

Cwikel, A., & Blit-Cohen, E. (2018). Strategies used by activists in Israeli environmental struggles: Implications for the future green social worker. In L. Dominelli (Ed.), *The Routledge handbook of green social work* (pp. 442–453). New York, NY: Routledge.

Dalin, C., Hanasaki, N., Qiu, H., Mauzerall, D. L., & Rodriguez-Iturbe, I. (2014). Water resource transfers through Chinese interprovincial and foreign food trade. *PNAS, 111*, 9774–9779. doi:10.1073/pnas.1404749111

Damschroder, L. J., Aron, D. C., Keith, R. E., Kirsh, S. R., Alexander, J. A., & Lowery, J. C. (2009). Fostering implementation of health services research findings into practice: A consolidated framework for advancing implementation science. *Implementation Science, 4*, 50. doi:10.1186/1748-5908-4-50

Despard, M. R., Ansong, D., Nafziger-Mayegun, R. N., & Adjabeng, B. (2018). Predictors of capacity-building needs among nongovernmental organizations in Sub-Saharan Africa. *Journal of Community Practice, 26*, 204–224. doi:10.1080/10705422.2018.1449043

Doering-White, J. (2018). Evidencing violence and care along the Central American Migrant Trail through Mexico. *Social Service Review, 92*, 432–469. doi:10.1086/699196

Dominelli, L. (2013). Environmental justice at the heart of social work practice: Greening the profession. *International Journal of Social Welfare, 22*, 431–439. doi:10.1111/ijsw.2013.22.issue-4

Dominelli, L. (2018). Green social work in theory and practice: A new environmental paradigm for the profession. In L. Dominelli (Ed.), *The Routledge handbook of green social work* (pp. 9–20). New York, NY: Routledge.

Droppa, D. C., & Giunta, C. (2015). Factors in the failure of seemingly successful human service collaboratives. *Human Service Organizations: Management, Leadership, & Governance, 39*, 125–138.

Eriksson, M., & Bjerge, B. (2019). Negotiating the social work profession. *Nordic Social Work Research, 9*, 1–4. doi:10.1080/2156857X.2019.1568370

Ferraro, F., Etzion, D., & Gehman, J. (2015). Tackling Grand Challenges pragmatically: Robust action revisited. *Organization Studies, 36*, 363–390. doi:10.1177/0170840614563742

George, G., Howard-Grenville, J., Joshi, A., & Thanyi, L. (2014). Understanding and tackling Grand Challenges through management research. *Academy of Management Journal, 59*, 1880–1895. doi:10.5465/amj.2016.4007

Ginwright, S. (2015). *Hope and healing in urban education: How urban activists and teachers are reclaiming matters of the heart*. New York, NY: Routledge.

Gummer, B. (1997). Organizational identity in a changing environment: When is a change a transformation? *Human Service Organizations: Management, Leadership, & Governance, 21*, 169–187.

Harlow, E., Berg, E., Barry, J., & Chandler, J. (2013). Neoliberalism, managerialism and the reconfiguring of social work in Sweden and the United Kingdom. *Organization, 20*, 534–550. doi:10.1177/1350508412448222

Hasenfeld, Y., & Garrow, E. E. (2012). Nonprofit human-service organizations, social rights, and advocacy in a neoliberal welfare state. *Social Service Review, 86*, 295–322. doi:10.1086/666391

Howard-Grenville, J., Buckle, S., Hoskins, B., & George, G. (2014). Climate change and management. *Academy of Management Journal, 57*, 615–623. doi:10.5465/amj.2014.4003

Intergovernmental Panel on Climate Change (IPCC). (2018). *Summary for policymakers. In: Global warming of 1.5°C. An IPCC Special Report on the impacts of global warming of 1.5°C above pre-industrial levels and related global greenhouse gas emission pathways, in the context of strengthening the global response to the threat of climate change, sustainable development, and efforts to eradicate poverty*. Geneva, Switzerland: World Meteorological Organization.

Kapucu, N., & Kuotsai, T. L. (2014). *Disaster and development: Examining global issues and cases*. New York, NY: Springer.

Karpouzoglou, T., Dewulf, A., & Clark, J. (2016). Advancing adaptive governance of social-ecological systems through theoretical multiplicity. *Environmental Science & Policy, 57*, 1–9. doi:10.1016/j.envsci.2015.11.011

Kearns, K. P. (2006). Faith-based and secular social service agencies in Pittsburgh: Location, mission, and organizational capacity. *Journal of Community Practice, 14*, 51–69. doi:10.1300/J125v14n04_04

Kemp, S. P., & Palinkas, L. A. (2015). *Strengthening the social response to the human impacts of environmental change*. Grand Challenges for Social Work Initiative Working Paper No. 5. American Academy of Social Work and Social Welfare.

Kim, H., & Zakour, M. (2018). Exploring the factors associated with the disaster preparedness of human service organizations serving persons with disabilities. *Human Service Organizations: Management, Leadership & Governance, 42*, 19–32.

Krings, A., Victor, B. G., Mathias, J., & Perron, B. E. (In press). Environmental social work in the disciplinary literature, 1991-2015. *International social work*.

Lok, J. (2019). Why (and how) institutional theory *can* be critical: Addressing the challenge to institutional theory's critical turn. *Journal of Management Inquiry, 28*, 335–349. doi:10.1177/1056492617732832

Maglaglic, R. A. (2019). Organization and delivery of social services in extreme events: Lessons from social work research on natural disasters. *International Social Work, 62*, 1146–1158. doi:10.1177/0020872818768387

Mason, L. R., & Rigg, J. (2019). Moving forward for community inclusion and policy change. In L. R. Mason & J. Rigg (Eds.), *People and climate change: Vulnerability, adaptation, and social justice* (pp. 211–218). New York, NY: Oxford University Press.

Mason, L. R., Shires, M. K., Arwood, C., & Borst, A. (2017). Social work research and global environmental change. *Journal of the Society for Social Work and Research, 8,* 645–671. doi:10.1086/694789

Mathias, J. (2018). Scales of value: Insiders and outsiders in environmental organizing in South India. *Social Service Review, 91,* 621–651. doi:10.1086/695352

McBeath, B. (2015). Making sense of HUSK: Practice implications for social change initiatives. *Journal of Evidence-Informed Social Work, 12,* 139–154.

McBeath, B., Mosley, J., Hopkins, K., Guerrero, E., Austin, M., & Tropman, J. E. (2019). Building knowledge to support human service organizational and management practice: An agenda to address the research-to-practice gap. *Social Work Research, 43,* 115–128. doi:10.1093/swr/svz003

McGurty, E. M. (1997). From NIMBY to civil rights: the origins of the environmental justice movement. *Environmental History, 2,* 301–323. doi: 10.2307/3985352

Moezzi, M., Janda, K. B., & Rotmann, S. (2017). Using stories, narratives, and storytelling in energy and climate change research. *Energy Research and Social Science, 31,* 1–10. doi:10.1016/j.erss.2017.06.034

Moldavanova, A., & Goerdel, H. T. (2018). Understanding the puzzle of organizational sustainability: Toward a conceptual framework of organizational social connectedness and sustainability. *Public Management Review, 20,* 55–81. doi:10.1080/14719037.2017.1293141

Mor Barak, M. (In press). The practice and science of social good: Emerging paths to positive social impact. *Research on Social Work Practice.*

Mosley, J. E. (2012). Keeping the lights on: How government funding concerns drive the advocacy agendas of nonprofit homeless service providers. *Journal of Public Administration Research and Theory, 22,* 841–866. doi:10.1093/jopart/mus003

Mosley, J. E. (2014). Collaboration, public-private intermediary organizations, and the transformation of advocacy in the field of homeless services. *American Review of Public Administration, 44,* 291–308. doi:10.1177/0275074012465889

Mulroy, E. A. (2004). Theoretical perspectives on the social environment to guide management and community practice: An organization-in-environment approach. *Human Service Organizations: Management, Leadership, & Governance, 28,* 77–96.

National Environmental Health Partnership Council. (2016). *The value of environmental health services: Exploring the evidence.* Washington, DC: American Public Health Association.

Nipperess, S., & Boddy, J. (2018). Greening Australian social work practice and education. In L. Dominelli (Ed.), *The Routledge handbook of green social work* (pp. 547–557). New York, NY: Routledge.

Orach, K., & Schlüter, M. (2016). Uncovering the political dimension of social-ecological systems: Contributions from policy process frameworks. *Global Environmental Change, 40,* 13–25. doi:10.1016/j.gloenvcha.2016.06.002

Philip, D., & Reisch, M. (2015). Rethinking social work's interpretation of 'environmental justice': From local to global. *Social Work Education, 34,* 471–483. doi:10.1080/02615479.2015.1063602

Powers, M. C. F., Willett, J., Mathias, J., & Hayward, A. (2018). Green social work for environmental justice: Implications for international social workers. In L. Dominelli (Ed.), *The Routledge handbook of green social work* (pp. 74–84). New York, NY: Routledge.

Ramsay, S., & Boddy, J. (2017). Environmental social work: A concept analysis. *British Journal of Social Work, 47,* 68–86.

Ramsundarsingh, S., & Shier, M. L. (2019). Anti-oppressive organizational dynamics in the social services: A literature review. *British Journal of Social Work, 47,* 2308–2327.

Reid, W. V., Chen, D., Goldfarb, L., Hackmann, H., Lee, Y. T., & Whyte, A. (2010). Earth system science for global sustainability: Grand challenges. *Science, 330,* 916–917. doi:10.1126/science.1196263

Reisch, M. (2019). *Macro social work practice: Working for change in a multicultural society.* San Diego, CA: Cognella.

Robinson, D. T. (2007). Control theories in sociology. *Annual Review of Sociology, 33,* 157–174. doi:10.1146/annurev.soc.32.061604.123110

Rousseau, D. M., & Gunia, B. C. (2016). Evidence-based practice: The psychology of EBP implementation. *Annual Review of Psychology, 67,* 667–692. doi:10.1146/annurev-psych-122414-033336

Schmid, H. (2004). Organization-environment relationships: Theory for management practice in human service organizations. *Human Service Organizations: Management, Leadership, & Governance, 28,* 97–113.

Schmid, H. (2019). Rethinking organizational reforms in human service organizations: Lessons, dilemmas, and insights. *Human Service Organizations: Management, Leadership, & Governance, 43,* 54–66.

Sharma-Wallace, L., Velarde, S. J., & Wreford, A. (2018). Adaptive governance good practice: Show me the evidence! *Journal of Environmental Management, 222,* 174–184. doi:10.1016/j.jenvman.2018.05.067

Shier, M. L., & Handy, F. (2015). From advocacy to social innovation: A typology of social change efforts by nonprofits. *Voluntas, 26,* 2581–2603. doi:10.1007/s11266-014-9535-1

Simo, G., & Bies, A. L. (2007). The role of nonprofits in disaster response: An expanded model of cross-sector collaboration. *Public Administration Review, 67,* 125–142. doi:10.1111/puar.2007.67.issue-s1

Smith, S. L. (2012). Coping with disaster: Lessons learned from executive directors of nonprofit organizations (NPOs) in New Orleans following Hurricane Katrina. *Human Service Organizations: Management, Leadership, & Governance, 36,* 359–389.

Stouten, J., Rousseau, D., & De Cremer, D. (2018). Successful organizational change: Integrating the management practice and scholarly literatures. *Academy of Management Annals, 12,* 752–788. doi:10.5465/annals.2016.0095

Teixeira, S., & Krings, A. (2015). Sustainable social work: An environmental justice framework for social work education. *Social Work Education, 34,* 513–527. doi:10.1080/02615479.2015.1063601

Thornton, P. H., Ocasio, W., & Lounsbury, M. (2012). *The institutional logics perspective: A new approach to culture, structure, and process.* New York, NY: Oxford University Press.

United Nations Human Rights Council (UNHRC). (2019, June 29). *Climate change and poverty.* Report of the Special Rapporteur on extreme poverty and human rights. Report A/HRC/41/39.

US Global Change Research Program. (2018). *Impacts, risks, and adaptation in the United States: Fourth national climate assessment, volume II: Report-in-brief.* Washington, DC: US Government Publishing Office.

Vangen, S., Hayes, J. P., & Cornforth, C. (2015). Governing cross-sector, inter-organizational collaborations. *Public Management Review, 17,* 1237–1260. doi:10.1080/14719037.2014.903658

Wang, Y. W., Liu, T., & Dang, H. (2018). Bridging critical institutionalism and fragmented authoritarianism in China: An analysis of centralized water policies and their local implementation in semi-arid irrigation districts. *Regulation & Governance, 12,* 451–465. doi:10.1111/rego.12198

Watson, L. D., & Hegar, R. L. (2013). The tri-sector environment of social work administration: Applying theoretical orientations. *Human Service Organizations: Management, Leadership, & Governance, 37,* 215–226.

Willett, J. (2019). Micro disasters: Expanding the social work conceptualization of disasters. *International Social Work, 62,* 133–145. doi:10.1177/0020872817712565

Willging, C. E., Gunderson, L., Green, A. E., Jaramillo, E. T., Garrison, L., Ehrhart, M. G., & Aarons, G. A. (2018). Perspectives from community-based organizational managers on implementing and sustaining evidence-based interventions in child welfare. *Human Service Organizations: Management, Leadership & Governance, 42,* 359–379.

Wright, C., & Nyberg, D. (2017). An inconvenient truth: How organizations translate climate change into business as usual. *Academy of Management Journal, 60,* 1633–1661. doi:10.5465/amj.2015.0718

Xu, Y., Ramanathan, V., & Victor, D. G. (2018). Global warming will happen faster than we think. *Nature, 564,* 30–32. doi:10.1038/d41586-018-07586-5

Yan, M. C., Cheung, J. C. S., Tsui, M. S., & Chu, C. K. (2017). Examining the neoliberal discourse of accountability: The case of Hong Kong's social service sector. *International Social Work, 60,* 976–989. doi:10.1177/0020872815594229

Social Good Science and Practice: A New Framework for Organizational and Managerial Research in Human Service Organizations

Michàlle E. Mor Barak

ABSTRACT

Volatile economic, demographic and political trends have severe implications for human service organizations (HSOs). Restricted governmental budgets threaten HSOs' funding and negative attitudes toward science threaten HSOs' evidence-based practices. A ray of light in this bleak context is the emergence of the *social good* movement that coalesces grassroots organizations, NGOs, governmental agencies, businesses, and philanthropists who are motivated to improve the lives of others. *Social good* refers to "individual, community and societal well-being in the domains of environmental justice, inclusion, and peace, achieved by engaging unconventional systems and utilizing innovative technologies, aiming to promote social justice". This paper: (a) examines contextual social forces challenging HSOs; (b) defines social good and its theoretical underpinnings; (c) presents an original model of social good and its relevance to HSOs; (d) introduces a framework for guiding future research in HSOs; and, (e) examines implications for practices, policies, and future research.

Volatile economic trends, mass immigration, and negative reactions to globalization over the past decade have served as an important contextual backdrop to human service organizations and have presented serious challenges for social work management (Kriesi & Pappas, 2015; Mor Barak, 2018a; Peters, 2017). These economic and demographic trends in the United States and around the world gave rise to populist movements[1] that have emerged during the second decade of the 21st century (Aslanidis, 2016; Mudde, 2004; Mudde & Kaltwasser, 2013). Recent developments go hand in hand with arguing for small government, less entitlements, challenging the elites, and questioning scientific data (Ostiguy & Roberts, 2016; Schindler, 2017). The implications for human service organizations have been grave for two reasons. First, restricted governmental budgets threaten HSOs' funding and therefore their ability to continue providing valuable services to populations in need. And, second, negative attitudes toward science in general, and research-based decision making in particular, present a threat to important efforts by human service organizations in recent decades to implement evidence-based practices (Aarons, Sommerfeld, Hecht, Silovsky, & Chaffin, 2009; Beidas et al., 2013).

A ray of light in this bleak context has been the emergence of a movement for *social good*. There is a burgeoning consciousness about the importance of "making a difference" and "contributing to society" that brings together previously unlikely collaborations between business organizations, individual citizens, celebrities, media outlets, philanthropists and grassroots organizations (Feldmann, 2016; Mor

---

Color versions of one or more of the figures in the article can be found online at www.tandfonline.com/wasw.

[1]For a definition of populism, see Mudde and Kaltwasser (2013), and Mudde (2004) who defines populism as "a thin-centered ideology that considers society to be ultimately separated into two homogeneous and antagonistic groups, 'the pure people' versus 'the corrupt elite', and which argues that politics should be an expression of the *volonté générale* (general will) of the people" (p. 543).

Barak, 2018b). The term *social good* refers, very broadly, to services or products that promote human well-being on a large scale (Business Dictionary, 2017). Services or products may include providing timely access to health care services, increasing educational attainment, improving equality and women's rights, and providing clean water and safe environment. Although the term social good and the initiatives to promote it have emerged organically from grassroots organizations and businesses, they embody ideals that are at the heart of the social work profession and that promote its core values and goals (Foley & Chowdhury, 2007; Verdugo, 2013; Viswanathan, Seth, Gau, & Chaturvedi, 2009). Social good initiatives have brought new perspectives, potential collaborators, and increased energy into finding innovative solutions for large-scale social causes, many of which are included in the social work profession's Grand Challenges statement (American Academy of Social Work and Social Welfare, 2017).

The social good movement represents a great promise for human service organizations as it could provide alternative sources of funding, an engagement of new volunteers, and strong support for the application of scientific knowledge to promote positive social change. This paper explores the social good movement and its potential relevance and applicability for human service organizational and managerial research. Specifically, the paper: (a) examines the contextual social forces that present challenges for human services organizations; (b) explores the social good movement and its relevance for human service organizations; and, (c) presents a framework for guiding future human service organizational and managerial research.

Contextual forces challenging human service organizations

The global economy is still reeling from the impact of the 2008 economic crisis and many nations are going through periods of economic upheaval. Some nations are experiencing a period of precarious economic prosperity coupled with high national debt (such as the U.S.), while others are going through economic volatility (e.g., some African and South American countries) and even being compelled to enforce austerity conditions (e.g., some European countries) (Addabbo et al., 2015; Arechavala, Espina, & Trapero, 2015). The economic uncertainty, particularly prosperity that has left large segments of society behind, has brought forth populist movements and leaders who publicly reject the "conventional" social order. Yet, these leaders have not been successful in delivering better living conditions to populations such as minorities, immigrants, and members of society who live in lower economic class communities (Inglehard & Norris, 2016). In recent years, the populism phenomenon has gained strength and reach in many countries and have had implications for social work and social policy in the U.S. and around the world (Fischer & Dunn, 2019; Kriesi & Pappas, 2015; Lockwood, 2018). Examples include the 2016 Brexit referendum in the UK, the 2016 election of Donald J. Trump in the USA, the 2017 strong performances by the Front National in the French Presidential election and Alternative für Deutschland (AfD) in the German general election, and the 2019 election of Boris Johnson as prime minister of the UK (Fischer & Dunn, 2019; Lockwood, 2018).

These global and national trends affect human service organizations in two ways. The first is the impact on their budgets. An integral part of populism is the rejection of "big government" and "big bureaucracies", which also means less funding for entitlement programs and social services (Ketola & Nordensvard, 2018). Because a significant proportion of HSOs' funding comes from governmental agencies, limited governmental spending has a significant impact on their budgets and on their ability to provide services to their clients. A second characteristic of populist movements is the rejection of "social elites". Scholars, researchers, and academics are often perceived as elites; and their products – scientific publications and data-driven research – are viewed with skepticism or even outright hostility (see, for example, climate change science, Lockwood, 2018). This trend presents a threat to human service organizations, which have worked hard over the past few decades to establish scientific evidence-based practices (see, for example, Aarons et al., 2009; Beidas et al., 2013; Ehrhart, Aarons, & Farahnak, 2014).

Social good – Relevance for human service organizations

The movement for social good[2] has emerged in the past decade, fueled by a sense of urgency around three broad societal challenges: economic and social inequalities, climate change and its environmental impact, and the need to address intergroup tensions and wars (for analysis of information gleaned from academic publications, Internet discourse, and qualitative interviews, see Mor Barak, 2018b). The quest to promote social good in the U.S. and around the world has brought together physical and virtual communities that have united around a cause or an idea, discoursing globally and instantaneously, and translating their concerns into coordinated actions (Feldmann, 2016). Among the actions to promote social good were protests or petition drives, organized through a combination of on-line social networks and on the ground actions. Prime examples of this phenomenon are the Black Lives Matter movement (Rickford, 2015) and the #OscarSoWhite protest against racial inequality in the Hollywood film industry (USA Today Feb. 2, 2016).

Broadly, the term *social good* refers to services or products that promote human well-being on a large scale (e.g., Business Dictionary, 2017). The following is a multi-dimensional definition, based on a state-of-the-art review of the literature and expert interviews (see Figure 1).

"*Social good* refers to individual, community and society well-being related to:
(a) Addressing three specific domains – environmental justice and sustainability, diversity and inclusion, and peace, harmony and collaboration;
(b) Engaging unconventional systems of change such as grassroots and business collaborations, national and international NGOs, and social entrepreneurs; and,
(c) Utilizing innovative technologies and approaches, such as design thinking, big data–driven models, and harnessing social media for social change.
All aiming to promote social justice." (Mor Barak, 2018b, p. 8).

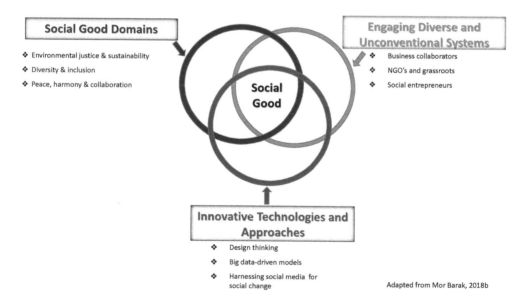

Figure 1. Defining Social Good.

Social good is a relatively new term and, therefore, requires some differential clarification to specify its difference from similarly sounding terms – *public goods* and *common goods* (Mor Barak, 2018b). The term *public goods* refers to products and services that are typically provided by the state or the federal government and is funded by taxation. These include services and products such as national defense, education, health services, and emergency services (Scott, 2014). In contrast, *social good* does not depend on public policy or public funding and typically draws on resources from several seemingly disparate systems, such as grassroots organizations, businesses, and social entrepreneurs. The second term, *common goods*, refers to voluntarily shared resources, which people manage by negotiating their own rules through social or customary traditions, norms and practices for the fulfillment of their needs (Melé, 2009; Messner, 1965). In contrast, *social good* is not tied to a specific community's goals, norms or resources and is often national or global in its aspirations, reach and resources.

Applications of the social good model to social work practice, policy, and to management of HSOs have emerged in recent years, combining several aspects of the social good model and demonstrating the importance of crossing systems boundaries and creating new alliances. In the area of environmental justice, for example, a longitudinal quasi-experimental pilot project has demonstrated the positive impact of participating in a recycling program that transforms reusable bottles into eco-friendly blankets for disaster survivors on older adults' psychological and physiological health (Hsiao et al., 2019). This program combined two areas of social good – environmental justice and diversity and inclusion – to create a positive impact for the environment (recycling), for environmental disaster survivors (providing eco-friendly blankets), and inclusion (of older adults). The program has also enlisted unconventional partnerships between senior centers, a community-based religious organization (Tzu Chi Foundation), and a for-profit business (DA.AI Technology). Their combined efforts contributed to social good for the older adult program participants, for their communities, and for disaster hit areas around the world (Hsiao et al., 2019).

A second example of the social good model is a qualitative study examining the benefits of providing mental health services to an immigrant community through an unconventional collaboration with a consulate (Helu-Brown & Barrio, 2019). The program, Modulo de Salud Mental, demonstrates an original way of overcoming structural and cultural barriers for service utilization by a Latino immigrant community. Rather than delivering the services in a traditional way through an HSO, the program created a collaboration with a Mexican consulate in the United States to deliver the services within the consulate. Findings suggest that the program's services that were delivered in an environment that was considered safe and trustworthy (the Mexican Consulate) significantly increased service utilization. This program can serve as a model for forging unconventional collaborations to facilitate help seeking behaviors in a minority community, improving inclusion and promoting social good (Helu-Brown & Barrio, 2019).

A third and most interesting example is in the social good model's domain of peace and reconciliation. It demonstrates the important role that Non-Governmental Organizations (NGOs) play in working toward social good (Almog-Bar, Cnaan, Pitowski-Nave, & Tury, 2019). The social work profession's involvement in the field of peace and co-existence is still limited and peripheral to the profession. Peace and coexistence should be a social work mainstay and be an integral part of social work curricula and discourse. Jane Addams, widely considered the founder of the social work profession, worked tirelessly to promote peace. In recognition of her efforts, she was the first American woman to win the Nobel Peace Prize in 1931 (Knight, 2005). Yet, the social work profession has abandoned some of Addams's ideals and few social workers have been involved in this field in recent decades (Johnson, 2004), which is essential for protecting human rights and supporting clients' well-being. Research indicates that successful international human service organizations are those who, in addition to focusing on social meetings between people from different sides, are working diligently toward peace and coexistence through understanding the power dynamics between the powerful and powerless sides of conflicts (Almog-Bar et al., 2019).

Social good coalesces many movements in the United States and around the world and unites different sectors of society – nonprofit, grassroots groups, philanthropists, businesses and international groups such as the United Nations. For example, the Social Good Summit, an annual conference focused on promoting social good around the world, is co-sponsored by the United Nations Foundation and businesses such as UBS, Facebook, and Pfizer (United Nations Foundation, 2018). In the past decades, we have seen different populations groups, such as university students, older adults, and schoolchildren engage in fundraising and activism to support causes in their communities, in their nations, and across the globe (Mohanty, 2010; Slocum & Rhoads, 2009). Research on millennials and post-millennials indicates that these generations are increasingly motivated to contribute to social good (e.g., Hershatter & Epstein, 2010; Leveson & Joiner, 2014; Meister & Willyerd, 2010; Ng & Gossett, 2013; Suleman & Nelson, 2011).

The social good movement is highly relevant to human service organizations and to the profession because it promotes ideals that directly align with the values and ethical obligations of the social work profession (Foley & Chowdhury, 2007; Verdugo, 2013; Viswanathan et al., 2009). It holds promise for creating alliances between social work and like-minded disciplines, businesses, grassroots organizations and philanthropic institutions. It has the potential for opening up new strategies and collaborations for social change, while also connecting with diverse constituencies and offering innovative solutions to pressing social problems. Social good is relevant to the mission of human service organizations as agents of social change, following the ideals articulated by Jane Addams (1893). Championing social good initiatives for the social work profession may accelerate the development of robust new theoretical models, research initiatives, and evidence-based practices that will stimulate renewed interest in the macro practice specialization, in the management of HSO, and in the Grand Challenges of the profession (American Academy of Social Work & Social Welfare, 2017).

Social good – Theoretical underpinning

Two theories have been suggested for explaining and describing cause and effect connections related to social good: social capital theory and virtue theory (Garlington, Collins, & Durham Bossaller, 2019; Mor Barak, 2018b). Social capital theory's main proposition is that individuals obtain resources through their networks of trusted social relationships (Coleman, 1988). The term social capital refers to "the sum of the actual and potential resources embedded within, available through, and derived from the network of relationships possessed by an individual or social unit" (Nahapiet & Ghoshal, 1998, p. 243). The theory can explain behaviors that address social problems on a large scale by incorporating advanced technologies, such as virtual communities that are focused on contributing to social good (Mor Barak, 2018b). Applying social capital theory to social good can demonstrate that online communities, for example, can increase the social capital of individuals and groups who unite around a social cause, enabling them to combine resources (e.g., ideas, funding, tools) and find solutions to social problems on a large scale (Briones, Kuch, Liu, & Jin, 2011; Lovejoy & Saxton, 2012).

The second theory proposed for explaining social good is virtue theory (Garlington et al., 2019). Aristotle and St. Thomas Aquinas developed the foundations for virtue theory in ancient times, among others, with contemporary contributions from scholars such as MacIntyre (1981). The theory focuses on the qualities of individuals and society that lead to human flourishing and thus connects social work to a long study of individual behavior and social dynamics (Collins, Cooney, & Garlington, 2012; Collins & Garlington, 2017; Collins, Garlington, & Cooney, 2015). Virtue theory can provide an analytical framework that links social good to the core values of the social work profession as well as to a range of allied disciplines. Particularly relevant to the study of social good is the theory's virtue of solidarity as it explains issues that are germane to the social good model such as mutual interest and recognition of human dignity (Garlington et al., 2019). For example, social inclusion and peaceful collaboration are components of solidarity and applying this element of virtue theory to social good creates a link to compassion and justice. As Clark (2014) notes, social inclusion, social cohesion, collaboration, or other bonding social capital measures could be exclusionary and reinforce oppressive power relationships if participating communities are unequal and if historical contexts are unexamined. A virtue theory framework, specifically the example of solidarity, facilitates a greater understanding of inequalities and power dynamics within a social good domain.

Social capital theory and virtue theory could serve as the foundations for developing a more robust theoretical framework for social good. Scholars will need to invest in additional theoretical work in order to explain these complex phenomena. Future theoretical development should focus on providing a more comprehensive theoretical approach that would be able to undergird the main concepts and mechanisms that are united under the term social good.

A social good framework for guiding future research in human service organizational and management

The social good movement presents a rare opportunity for social work researchers to be at the forefront of this emerging area of scientific inquiry. It is particularly relevant to HSOs and to social work managers because social good involves working within organizations and collaborating across systems with other organizations and entities such as businesses, grassroots organizations, and volunteers. A review of the literature indicates that academia has lagged behind in addressing social good, using the construct primarily as a contextual descriptor or referring broadly to the social phenomenon (Mor Barak, 2018b), thus opening up opportunities for interdisciplinary inquiry led by social work researchers. There is clearly a need to explore social good from interdisciplinary perspectives and to propose a scientific agenda for the social work profession that will amplify its potential for impact in promoting social justice.

The National Science Foundation (NSF) defines convergence science as *an approach to problem solving that cuts across disciplinary boundaries* (National Science Foundation, 2017). The NSF characterizes convergence science as the deep integration of knowledge, techniques, and expertise from multiple fields to form new and expanded frameworks for addressing scientific and societal challenges and opportunities (NSF, 2017). According to the NSF's definition, by merging diverse areas of expertise in a network of partnerships, convergence stimulates innovation from basic science discovery to translational application. Research into the broad challenges associated with generating social good in our society will require deep transdisciplinary partnerships and could potentially lead to the development of convergence collaborations.

Social good is challenging practitioners and scholars alike to think big about solutions to social problems, to use new avenues for social change, such as technology and social media, and to open the door to innovative partnerships and collaborative models. There is promising synergy between the social good movement and the mission and values of the social work profession. We need to understand how to leverage this synergy through future research that would explore new collaborative practice models for social work management and for HSOs.

Given its history and goals, the social work profession can be a leader in scholarship as well as the practical applications of social good. Accordingly, the future research agenda for human service organizations and management needs to focus on five major areas (depicted in Figure 2):

(1) **Develop theoretical frameworks** for promoting social good in organizations and society. This will include developing theoretical models for understanding organizational and individual motivation for engaging in activities leading to social good, understanding avenues for creativity and innovation in social good, and intergenerational engagement and collaborations related to social good affecting positive outcomes of such activities for individuals, organizations and communities. Examples include using virtue theory and the concept of solidarity to connect social good to social work professional values (Garlington et al., 2019) and reexamining social justice in the context of modern societies and post-modern knowledge in order to define the kinds of social justice that the social good movement should aspire to (Levin, 2019).

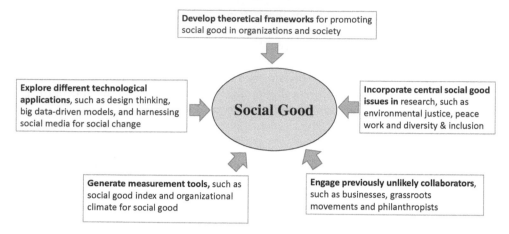

Figure 2. Future social good research for management and human service organizations.

(2) **Incorporate central social good issues in research**. Research questions could include ways for incorporating the social good domains of environmental justice, peace and intergroup relations, and diversity and inclusion into the core activities of human service organizations. Such research would examine avenues to accomplish environmental justice for local communities, engage in intergroup dialog related to peace and reconciliation both nationally and internationally, and conduct research that examines inclusion among diverse communities as well as within human service organizations themselves. Studies could focus on adding the often-overlooked issue of environmental justice to the activities of human service organizations through collaborations with other organizations (Kemp & Palinkas, 2015). An example of working with communities to accomplish environmental justice could include engaging adults and children in citizen science activities (lay people working under the guidance of professional scientists) to collect samples of contaminated water or soil in their homes such as in the case of the Flint, Michigan water contamination disaster (Markuch & Aczel, 2019).

(3) **Engage previously unlikely collaborators**, such as businesses, grassroots movements and philanthropists in the work of HSOs around the common goal of promoting social good. With the prospect of limited governmental spending on welfare services and the looming financial distress for human service organizations, research in this area could focus on pilot testing initiatives that generate unconventional collaborations. For example, research could examine collaborations between HSOs and for-profit businesses, engaging volunteers from businesses in HSO activities, and engaging philanthropists and foundations in the work of the organization by contributing not only funds but also to ideas and initiatives (e.g., Helu-Brown & Barrio, 2019; Hsiao et al., 2019). Research questions could include, for example, comparing different engagement models for collaborations between HSOs and business organizations, how to engage business volunteers in promoting environmental justice for local communities, and how to effectively utilize social media experts in promoting social policies that benefit HSOs' clients.

(4) **Generate measurement tools**. It is important to create measurement scales to assess goal attainment with respect to social good. Such measures would include, for example, a social good index and a measure of organizational climate for social good. Just like organizational climates for safety, innovation, or inclusion, organizations could have a climate for social good. Broadly, organizational climate is defined as shared perceptions among members with respect to a specific issue (Mor Barak, 2017; Nishii, 2013; Shore et al., 2011; Zohar & Hofmann, 2012). In this case, climate for social good could include such items as the extent

to which members of the organization and management see value for employee engagement in activities that contribute to social good. It would also assess the extent to which the organization supports such activities by providing opportunities for participating in social good activities in the community or with philanthropic organizations and by giving release or paid time for these activities.

(5) **Explore different technological applications**. Researchers could focus on generating new initiatives and assessing existing ones to engage HSO employees and clients in collaborations utilizing data to improve services. Studies could examine different innovative applications of technology, such as design thinking, big data–driven models, and harnessing social media for social change. Research initiatives would focus on, for example, studying the potential of online communities to improve the well-being of clients and promote specific social policies. They could also examine the risks involved with using social media. Research could pose questions such as: How to utilize social networking platforms to raise awareness of social issues?; How to recruit volunteers through social networking sites to promote specific policies?; and, How to recruit business collaborators and volunteers with advanced technological skills to deliver social work services to populations that would otherwise not have access to these services? These research initiatives could test new technologies to deliver services to clients, to promote social policies, to improve the lives of community residents, and to create a sense of community.

Implications for practice in management and organizations

Social good has the potential to become an important element of social work practice in general and of macro practice in particular. It provides a strong link between the roots of the social work profession on the one hand, and its future aspirations on the other. Jane Addams, the founder of the social work profession, worked toward improving all three of the social good domains. Specifically, she promoted social inclusion of immigrant families and women, she worked toward peace and reconciliation, and she promoted environmental justice, advocating on behalf of the disadvantaged groups living in the tenements of Chicago surrounding Hull House (Johnson, 2004; Senecah, 2017; Steyaert, 2013). Social good is also strongly connected to the future aspirations of the social work profession as expressed through the Grand Challenges for Social Work (American Academy of Social Work & Social Welfare, 2017). Each of the twelve Grand Challenges requires engaging systems of collaboration and innovative technology, and together they all promote social good.

Macro social work practice emphasizes social change and consists of interventions with large systems that include communities, organizations, and society at large, focused on alleviating suffering and enacting social justice (Hill, Ferguson, & Erickson, 2010; McBeath & Webb, 2002; Rothman, 2013). Social good allows macro practitioners to expand the horizons of social work practice in communities and organizations and to include new forms and new domains. For example, promoting social good in the context of diverse HSOs inevitably involves finding ways for all organizational members to feel valued and appreciated for who they are by creating inclusive work environments (Brimhall & Saastamoinen, 2019; Mor Barak, 2017). Creating inclusive organizational climates is particularly important for leaders of HSOs at the top levels as well as middle managers and direct supervisors (Brimhall & Mor Barak, 2018; Mor Barak, 2015). It is important for managers to not only state the importance of diversity and inclusion for the organization, but also make sure that they implement inclusive practices at all levels of the organization. Similarly, inclusion for social good is relevant to addressing important social problems such as mass incarceration. The racially based systematic social exclusion in the United States has been the foundation of mass incarceration, particularly the over-incarceration of African Americans (Cox, 2019).

Another example provides a path toward improving environmental justice through involving children, particularly from disadvantaged communities, in citizen science, defined as science conducted by non-specialists under the direction of professional scientists (Markuch & Aczel, 2019).

Environmental justice includes notions of equality, equity, social inclusion, human rights, public participation, and accountability (Agyeman, Bullard, & Evans, 2002). HSOs can get involved with local businesses and academic institutes to coordinate and lead efforts to involve children, their families, and their communities in scientific efforts to examine and improve their own environment. These initiatives could include activities such as testing water and air qualities, reporting those results to local state and government authorities, and then organizing the community for action to make sure that improvements are implemented (Markuch & Aczel, 2019).

Conclusion

The potential centrality of social good to the mission and values of the social work profession is derived from its relationship to social justice with respect to shared overall goals. It also calls for collaborations with other disciplines such as management, health, education, and law (Banerjee, 2008; Bemak & Chung, 2005; Ginwright & James, 2002; Ruger, 2004). Social justice has long been central to professional and academic social work discourse (Craig, 2002; Dominelli, 2004; Ferguson, 2007; Levin, 2019). To some extent, the domains of social good – diversity and inclusion, environmental justice, and peace and intergroup collaborations – represent updated areas of social justice.

In conclusion, social good can open up new opportunities for the social work profession, together with allied sectors and disciplines, to lead the development of evidence-based practices and educational programs aimed at promoting social justice. Social good suggests the need for more expansive perspectives on systems of change for the social work profession. It carries new energy to the fight for social justice in its reliance on partnerships and cross-disciplinary or inter-disciplinary collaborations; its celebration of innovation and technology; and its support of macro solutions for social ills (Levin, 2019; Mor Barak, 2018b). It can bring a fresh perspective and direction to HSOs, rooted in the profession's bedrock values of social justice and befitting the entrepreneurial spirit and technological innovations of the 21st century.

Disclosure statement

No potential conflict of interest was reported by the author.

References

Aarons, G. A., Sommerfeld, D. H., Hecht, D. B., Silovsky, J. F., & Chaffin, M. J. (2009). The impact of evidence-based practice implementation and fidelity monitoring on staff turnover: Evidence for a protective effect. *Journal of Consulting and Clinical Psychology*, 77(2), 270–280. doi:10.1037/a0013223

Addabbo, T., Bastos, A., Casaca, S. F., Duvvury, N., & Ní Léime, Á. (2015). Gender and labour in times of austerity: Ireland, Italy and Portugal in comparative perspective. *International Labour Review*, 154, 449–473. doi:10.1111/j.1564-913X.2015.00250.x

Addams, J. (1893). The subjective necessity for social settlements. In J. Addams, R. A. Woods, J. O. S. Huntington, F. H. Giddings, & B. Bosanquet (Eds.), *Philanthropy and social progress: Seven essays* (pp. 1–26). New York, NY: T. Y. Crowell & Co.

Agyeman, J., Bullard, R. D., & Evans, B. (2002). Exploring the nexus: Bringing together sustainability, environmental justice and equity. *Space and Polity*, 6(1), 77–90. doi:10.1080/13562570220137907

Almog-Bar, M., Cnaan, R., Pitowski-Nave, N., & Tury, K. (2019). Coexistence and peace nonprofits in Israel promoting social good: Characteristics of active and inactive organizations. *Research on Social Work Practice*, (In Press) doi:10.1177/1049731519868010

American Academy of Social Work & Social Welfare. (2017). *Grand challenges for social work*. The American Academy of Social Work and Social Welfare. Retrieved from http://aaswsw.org/grand-challenges-initiative/

Arechavala, N. S., Espina, P. Z., & Trapero, B. P. (2015). The economic crisis and its effects on the quality of life in the European Union. *Social Indicators Research*, 120, 323–343. doi:10.1007/s11205-014-0595-9

Aslanidis, P. (2016). Populist Social Movements of the Great Recession. *Mobilization: An International Quarterly*, 21 (3), 301–321. doi:10.17813/1086-671X-20-3-301

Banerjee, S. B. (2008). Corporate social responsibility: The good, the bad and the ugly. *Critical Sociology*, *34*(1), 51–79. doi:10.1177/0896920507084623

Beidas, R. S., Aarons, G., Frances, B., Evans, A., Hadley, T., Hoagwood, K., & Mandell, D. (2013). Policy to implementation: Evidence-based practice in community mental health-Study protocol. *Implementation Science*, *8* (38), 1–9. doi:10.1186/1748-5908-8-38

Bemak, F., & Chung, R. C. Y. (2005). Advocacy as a critical role for urban school counsellors: Working toward equity and social justice. *Professional School Counselling*, *8*(3), 196–202.

Brimhall, K. C., & Mor Barak, M. E. (2018). The critical role of workplace inclusion in fostering innovation, job satisfaction, and quality of care in a diverse healthcare environment. *Human Service Organizations*, *5*(42), 474–492.

Brimhall, K. C., & Saastamoinen, M. (2019). Striving for social good through organizational inclusion: A latent profile approach. *Research on Social Work Practice, (First Published online)*. doi:10.1177/1049731519832103.

Briones, R. L., Kuch, B., Liu, B. F., & Jin, Y. (2011). Keeping up with the digital age: How the American red cross uses social media to build relationships. *Public Relations Review*, *37*, 37–43. doi:10.1016/j.pubrev.2010.12.006

Business Dictionary. (2017). *Social good*. Business Directory. Retrieved from http://www.businessdictionary.com/definition/social-good.html

Clark, M. J. (2014). *The vision of Catholic social thought: The virtue of solidarity & the praxis of human rights*. Minneapolis, MN: Fortress Press.

Coleman, J. S. (1988). Social capital in the creation of human capital. *American Journal of Sociology*, *94*, 95–120. doi:10.1086/228943

Collins, M. E., Cooney, K., & Garlington, S. (2012). Compassion in contemporary social policy: Applications of virtue theory. *Journal of Social Policy*, *41*, 251–269. doi:10.1017/S004727941100078X

Collins, M. E., & Garlington, S. (2017). Compassionate response: Intersections of religion & public policy. *Journal of Religion & Spirituality in Social Work*, *36*, 391–408.

Collins, M. E., Garlington, S., & Cooney, K. (2015). Relieving human suffering: Compassion in social policy. *Journal of Sociology & Social Welfare*, *48*, 95–120.

Cox, R. 2019. Applying the theory of social good to mass incarceration and civil rights, research on social work practice. First Published September 26, 2019. doi:10.1177/1049731519872838

Craig, G. (2002). Poverty, social work and social justice. *British Journal of Social Work*, *32*(6), 669–682. doi:10.1093/bjsw/32.6.669

Dominelli, L. (2004). *Social work: Theory and practice for a changing profession*. Bristol, UK: Polity Press.

Ehrhart, M. G., Aarons, G. A., & Farahnak, L. R. (2014). Assessing the organizational context for EBP implementation: The development and validity testing of the Implementation Climate Scale (ICS). *Implementation Science*, *9*(1), 157. doi:10.1186/s13012-014-0157-1

Feldmann, D. (2016). *Social movements for good: How companies and causes create viral change*. Hoboken, New Jersey, USA: John Wiley & Sons.

Ferguson, I. (2007). *Reclaiming social work: Challenging neo-liberalism and promoting social justice*. Thousand Oaks, CA: Sage.

Fischer, J., & Dunn, K. (Eds.). (2019). *Stifled progress – International perspectives on social work and social policy in the era of right-wing populism*. Berlin, Germany: Barbara Budrich Publishers.

Foley, D., & Chowdhury, J. (2007). Poverty, social exclusion and the politics of disability: Care as a social good and the expenditure of social capital in Chuadanga, Bangladesh. *Social Policy & Administration*, *41*, 372–385. doi:10.1111/j.1467-9515.2007.00559.x

Garlington, S. B., Collins, M. E., & Durham Bossaller, M. R. (2019). An ethical foundation for social good: Virtue theory and solidarity. *Research on Social Work Practice*, Published First on line. doi:10.1177/1049731519839472.

Ginwright, S., & James, T. (2002). From assets to agents of change: Social justice, organizing, and youth development. *New Directions for Youth Development*, *96*, 27–46. doi:10.1002/yd.25

Helu-Brown, P., & Barrio, C. (2019). Latinx mental health in the Mexican Consulate: Addressing barriers through social good. *Research on Social Work Practice*, (First Published, April 3). doi:10.1177/1049731519839465.

Hershatter, A., & Epstein, M. (2010). Millennials and the world of work: An organization and management perspective. *Journal of Business and Psychology*, *25*, 211–223. doi:10.1007/s10869-010-9160-y

Hill, K. M., Ferguson, S. M., & Erickson, C. (2010). Sustaining & strengthening a macro identity: The association of macro practice social work. *Journal of Community Practice*. doi:10.1080/10705422.2010.519684

Hsiao, H., Hsu, C., Chen, L., Wu, J., Chang, P., Line, C., … Lin, T. (2019). Effects of environmental volunteerism for social good on older adults' psychological and physiological well-being: A longitudinal quasi-experimental pilot study. *Research on Social Work Practice* ((In Print)).

Inglehard, R. F., & Norris, P. (2016). *Trump, Brexit, and the rise of populism: Economic have-nots and cultural backlash (July 29)*. HKS Working Paper No. RWP16-026. Retrieved from https://ssrn.com/abstract=2818659

Johnson, A. K. (2004). Social work is standing on the legacy of Jane Addams: But are we sitting on the sidelines? *Social Work*, *49*, 319–322.

Kemp, P. S., Palinkas, L. A., and Mason L. R. 2018 Create social responses to a changing environment. In R. Fong, J.E. Lubben and R. P Barth, Granc Challenges for Social Work and Society, New York, NY, USA: Oxford University Press.

Ketola, M., & Nordensvard, J. (2018). Reviewing the relationship between social policy and the contemporary populist radical right: Welfare chauvinism, welfare nation state and social citizenship. *Journal of International and Comparative Social Policy*, 34(3), 172–187. doi:10.1080/21699763.2018.1521863

Knight, L. W. (2005). *Citizen: Jane Addams and the struggle for democracy*. Chicago, IL: University of Chicago Press.

Kriesi, H., & Pappas, T. S. (Eds.). (2015). *European populism in the shadow of the great recession*. Colchester, London, UK: ECPR Press.

Leveson, L., & Joiner, A. T. (2014). Exploring corporate social responsibility values of millennial job-seeking students. *Education+ Training*, 56, 21–34. doi:10.1108/ET-11-2012-0121

Levin, L. (2019). Re-thinking social justice: A contemporary challenge for social good. *Research on Social Work Practice*, (First Published, June 12). doi:10.1177/1049731519854161.

Lockwood, M. (2018). Right-wing populism and the climate change agenda: Exploring the linkages. *Environmental Politics*, 27(4), 712–732. doi:10.1080/09644016.2018.1458411

Lovejoy, K., & Saxton, G. D. (2012). Information, community, and action: How nonprofit organizations use social media. *Journal of Computer-Mediated Communication*, 17, 337–353. doi:10.1111/j.1083-6101.2012.01576.x

MacIntyre, A. (1981). *After virtue*. Notre Dame, IN: University of Notre Dame Press.

Markuch, K. E., & Aczel, M. R. (2019). Environmental citizen science for social good: Engaging children and promoting justice, diversity, health and inclusion. *Research on Social Work Practice* ((In Press)).

McBeath, G., & Webb, S. A. (2002). Virtue ethics & social work: Being lucky, realistic, & not doing one's duty. *British Journal of Social Work*, 32, 1015–1036. doi:10.1093/bjsw/32.8.1015

Meister, J. C., & Willyerd, K. (2010). Mentoring millennials. *Harvard Business Review*, 88, 68–72.

Melé, D. (2009). Integrating personalism into virtue-based business ethics: The personalist and the common good principles. *Journal of Business Ethics*, 88, 227–244. doi:10.1007/s10551-009-0108-y

Messner, J. (1965). *Social ethics. Natural law in the Western World* (Revised ed.). St Louis, MO: B. Herder Book Co.

Mohanty, R. (2010). Contesting development, reinventing democracy: Grassroots social movements in India. In L. Thompson & C. Tapscott (Eds.), *Citizenship and social movements: Perspectives from the global south* (pp. 239–241). London, UK: Zed.

Mor Barak, M. E. (2015). Inclusion is the key to diversity management, but what *is* inclusion? (Guest Editorial). *Human Service Organizations: Management Leadership and Governance*, 39, 83–88. doi:10.1080/23303131.2015.1035599

Mor Barak, M. E. (2017). *Managing diversity: Toward a globally inclusive workplace* (4th ed.). Thousand Oaks, CA: Sage.

Mor Barak, M. E. (2018a). Erecting walls versus tearing them down: Inclusion and the (false) paradox of diversity in times of economic upheaval. *European Management Review*, 1–19. doi:10.1111/emre.12302

Mor Barak, M. E. (2018b). The practice and science of social good: Emerging paths to positive social impact. *Research on Social Work Practice*, 1–12. doi:10.1177/1049731517745600

Mudde, C. (2004). The populist Zeitgeist. *Government and Opposition*, 39(4), 541–563. doi:10.1111/j.1477-7053.2004.00135.x

Mudde, C., & Kaltwasser, C. R. (2013). Exclusionary vs. Inclusionary Populism: Comparing Contemporary Europe and Latin America. *Government and Opposition*, 48(2), 147–174. doi:10.1017/gov.2012.11

Nahapiet, J., & Ghoshal, S. (1998). Social capital, intellectual capital, and the organizational advantage. *Academy of Management Review*, 23, 242–266. doi:10.5465/amr.1998.533225

National Science Foundation. (2017) *Convergence research at NSF*. Author. Retrieved from https://www.nsf.gov/od/oia/convergence/index.jsp

Ng, E. S., & Gossett, C. W. (2013). Career choice in Canadian public service: An exploration of fit with the millennial generation. *Public Personnel Management*, 42, 337–358. doi:10.1177/0091026013495767

Nishii, L. H. (2013). The benefits of climate for inclusion for gender-diverse groups. *Academy of Management Journal*, 56, 1754–1774. doi:10.5465/amj.2009.0823

Ostiguy, P., & Roberts, K. M. (2016). Putting Trump in comparative perspective: Populism and the politicization of the sociocultural law. *The Brown Journal of World Affairs*, 23, 25.

Peters, M. A. (2017). The end of neoliberal globalisation and the rise of authoritarian populism. *Educational Philosophy and Theory*, The Education Philosophy and Theory. doi:10.1080/00131857.2017.1305720.

Rickford, R. (2015, December 8). Black lives matter: Toward a modern practice of mass struggle. *New Labor Forum*. doi:10.1177/1095796015620171

Rothman, J. (2013). *Education for macro intervention: A survey of problems & prospects*. Chicago, IL: Association for Community Organization and Social Administration.

Ruger, J. P. (2004). Health and social justice. *The Lancet*, 364(9439), 1075–1080. doi:10.1016/S0140-6736(04)17064-5

Schindler, F. (2017). Ignorant, stubborn, and unwilling to listen [MicroBusiness]. *IEEE Microwave Magazine*, 18, 22–27. doi:10.1109/MMM.2016.2636678

Scott, J. (2014). *A dictionary of sociology* (4th ed.). New York, NY: Oxford University Press.

Senecah, S. L. (2017). *1889 Jane Addams*. The History of Social Work. Retrieved from http://www.pollutionissues.com/A-Bo/Addams-Jane.html

Shore, L. M., Randel, A. E., Chung, B. G., Dean, M. A., Holcombe Ehrhart, K., & Singh, G. (2011). Inclusion and diversity in work groups: A review and model for future research. *Journal of Management, 37*, 1262–1289. doi:10.1177/0149206310385943

Slocum, J., & Rhoads, R. A. (2009). Faculty and student engagement in the Argentine grassroots rebellion: Toward a democratic and emancipatory vision of the university. *Higher Education, 57*, 85–105. doi:10.1007/s10734-008-9134-4

Steyaert, J. (2013). *Jane Addams: Settlement work in North America*. History of Social Work. Retrieved from http://www.historyofsocialwork.org/eng/details.php?canon_id=137

Suleman, R., & Nelson, B. (2011). Motivating the millennials: Tapping into the potential of the youngest generation. *Leader to Leader, 62*, 39–44. doi:10.1002/ltl.491

United Nations Foundation. (2018). Social good summit. Retrieved from https://unfoundation.org/event/social-good-summit-2018/

USA Today Feb. 2. (2016). *#OscarSoWhite controversy: What you need to know*. Retrieved from https://www.usatoday.com/story/life/movies/2016/02/02/oscars-academy-award-nominations-diversity/79645542/

Verdugo, R. R. (2013). School reform: Community, corporatism, and the social good. *International Journal of Educational Reform, 22*, 118. doi:10.1177/105678791302200201

Viswanathan, M., Seth, A., Gau, R., & Chaturvedi, A. (2009). Ingraining product-relevant social good into business processes in subsistence marketplaces: The sustainable market orientation. *Journal of Macromarketing, 29*, 406–425. doi:10.1177/0276146709345620

Zohar, D., & Hofmann, D. A. (2012). Organizational culture and climate. In S. W. J. Kozlowski (Ed.), *The Oxford handbook of organizational psychology* (Vol. 1, pp. 643–666). New York, NY: Oxford University Press.

How the "What Works" Movement is Failing Human Service Organizations, and What Social Work Can Do to Fix It

Jennifer E. Mosley ⓘ, Nicole P. Marwell, and Marci Ybarra

ABSTRACT

The social work profession has a long history of seeking legitimacy by adopting frameworks and methods from higher status professions. This quest has led to concerns about social work's strengths potentially being sacrificed for broader professional approval. In this commentary we explore a contemporary iteration of this phenomenon—social work's participation in the "What Works" movement, which promotes greater use of evidence-based practice (EBP) and policy—and discuss the impact of increasingly linking government funding for human service organizations (HSOs) to the use of EBPs. At risk are three foundations of social work practice: valuing community-based knowledge; preserving staff autonomy and a pipeline for social work trained managers; and making program decisions with a thorough understanding of organizational and community context. We argue that an organizational learning perspective may help HSOs maintain social work values while also drawing on evidence to improve the lives of consumers and their communities.

The history of social work is filled with stories of the field's struggles to be recognized as a legitimate, professional, and scientific enterprise. Abbott (1995) notes the precarious dependence of social work, situated on the boundaries of related, ultimately higher-status, professional fields, such as medicine and psychiatry. Deegan (1988) wrote of the late-19th century separation of sociology and social work, when the former claimed "scientific objectivity" while the latter was relegated to "do-gooderism." Stivers (2000) tells a similar story about the jointly emerging fields of social work and public administration in the Progressive Era, and how their different views of science and evidence led to very different outcomes for the two fields: for public administration, data was used to signal objectivity and efficiency, while for social work evidence was grounded in experiential connection to the meaningful change social workers sought in the world – a model that while contextually rich that was seen as less legitimate.

Social work's struggle to be recognized as "scientific" continues today. Specifically, we note the rise of a similar discourse about the value of "objective" evidence in current social work scholarship, with a growing share of social work scholars identifying as intervention and/or implementation scientists. This is part of the larger, interdisciplinary "What Works" movement populated by participants from economics, public policy, education, and more. It is an appealing approach and an important development for applied researchers who want their work to have a positive impact on people's lives.

But while we applaud efforts to ensure that social workers are delivering the highest quality programs to those who need them, we worry about social work losing some of its distinctive contributions – a fate that has befallen parallel professions. For instance, Stivers (2000) argues that in public administration, an inexorable shift occurred when the field went from simply conceptualizing science as a critical tool with which to push forward social reform goals, to focusing primarily on the technical details of scientific procedure. In other words, the legitimacy of science and data became an end in itself, with a concurrent decline in the actual ability of the field to produce significant social change.

In this short essay, we use social work's historical pursuit of scientific legitimacy as a jumping-off point to suggest the need for caution as intervention and implementation science become increasingly central in our field. These approaches typically assume social science – particularly experimental methods – to be a politically neutral endeavor focused on determining "what works" in social policy and programs. We argue instead that the focus on particular modes of evaluation and evidence may affect the field in ways that are not neutral at all.

As students of organizations, we feel compelled to ask whether the way this movement is playing out in social work is having unintended consequences on one of the most important tools we have to improve people's lives: human service organizations (hereafter HSOs). We do not advocate a rejection of science and evidence in social policy and programs. Determining what interventions have the most potential to help individuals, families, and communities in need is a laudable goal, and as social scientists ourselves, it is hard to take the position that there might be a downside to emphasizing science and evidence as the basis for decision-making and program development. But to achieve this, we contend that greater attention must be paid to the organizational settings in which such evidence is built, deployed, and ultimately replicated. In this essay we outline three major concerns about the movement for evidence-based policy and practice (hereafter EBP) in social work: 1) that valuable community-based knowledge may be sacrificed, potentially harming communities of color and marginalized groups, 2) that professional autonomy and leadership are increasingly under threat, and 3) that the organizational context of program implementation is systematically under-conceptualized and discounted. We then make the case for an alternative way of thinking about using evidence to improve social service delivery: a focus on organizational learning.

The role of community-based knowledge

One concern about the EBP movement is that it is fundamentally top-down in its orientation. The evidence in question is created, legitimated, and disseminated by elites, such as scholars, philanthropists, and federal funding bodies – not by local agencies or community members themselves. This sits in direct contradiction to social work's foundational value of self-determination, as well as decades of U.S. social policy that has aimed to involve grassroots interests in program and policy development and implementation. Conservatives and liberals alike have supported the idea that policy actors closer to communities – such as nonprofit HSOs – should be empowered to respond to the diverse needs and preferences of client populations and places. Indeed, the entire rationale for government support of nonprofit HSOs is that in a democracy as diverse as the U.S., public funds should go to a range of constituencies and support a large set of programs linked to those constituencies' unique needs (Salamon, 1995).

The EBP movement instead has moved to link government funding to pre-approved and standardized program models, arguing that it is irresponsible and perhaps unethical to direct taxpayer money to social programs that lack an evidence base. For example, the Family First Prevention Services Act of 2018 authorizes new federal funding for services aimed at families involved in the child welfare system, but only for programs that are registered and approved by the Title IV-E Prevention Services Clearinghouse. Another example is the Centers for Disease Control and Prevention's Diffusion of Effective Behavioral Interventions (DEBI) project, which prioritized and funded only specific interventions that had been rigorously evaluated in the treatment and prevention of HIV/AIDS. It is worth noting that, for example, this included pushing PrEP in communities of color in the South, where acceptance is lower and poverty is seen as a widespread and under-acknowledged social determinant of the disease (Green, 2018).

If federal, state, and local funding bodies choose to only fund programs that meet certain evidentiary criteria, then programs designed by people at the ground level and/or aimed at the most marginalized will find it increasingly difficult to gain government and foundation financial support. This is because small, community-based programs are unlikely to be able to mobilize the funds required to produce evidence, or to have the capacity to field research-based programs (Carman & Fredericks 2008). We argue this stance contradicts contemporaneous efforts to improve representation of marginalized groups in program development and delivery. Such small, community based programs also are more likely to serve specific populations – e.g., ethnic/racial or gender and sexual identity groups – often considered to be "ungeneralizable" to the common white, cis, straight "default" found in much evaluation research. This means programs designed by academic researchers and more elite organizations are the ones that stand to benefit most from experimental research regimes and related evidentiary ranking systems.

That said, we recognize that many social work interventionists have focused on developing interventions aimed at helping specific marginalized populations in culturally informed ways (Bouris et al., 2013; Hurdle, 2002; Spencer et al., 2011). This is an important reason why social work should be at the table as a key part of the EBP movement. While efforts to ensure representation and cultural humility in research are important, however, this approach does not fundamentally change the structure of the research industry (i.e., who pays for, develops, and carries out the interventions). As such, ground-level knowledge about how best to serve marginalized groups becomes marginalized in and of itself.

With government funds making up the vast majority of most HSOs' budgets (Boris, de Leon, Roeger, & Nikolova, 2010), the increased linkage of funds with the use of specific program models is likely to lead to one of two results. In one scenario, smaller organizations or those serving smaller population groups will be absorbed by larger organizations with the capacity and resources to implement evidence-based programs. In a second scenario, many of these smaller organizations will simply die out (only a few are likely to be able to survive on philanthropic support alone). Both scenarios are likely to result in a winnowing of programs that meet specialized needs, as well as decreased organizational program diversity in the human services sector.

It doesn't have to be this way. Leaders of the EBP movement promote an oft-cited three-circle model of evidence-based practice. One circle constitutes the best available evidence; another constitutes client or population values, preferences and needs; the third constitutes resources, including professional wisdom and expertise (Satterfield et al., 2009). Unfortunately, this "full" EBP model is not what usually happens on the ground when managers must adopt a specific program model to maintain their government funding or to qualify for certain initiatives. And even when adaptation of the research model is encouraged, HSOs will struggle with determining the degree of adaptation that is appropriate, rather than a violation of fidelity to a model. While the "full" EBP approach thus rightly focuses on context, culture, and existing assets as well as evidence, the ever-growing constraints placed on HSOs may hamper their ability to fully consider all these domains.

To achieve a future where diversity and autonomy are valued alongside research evidence, social work researchers – and managers at organizations where interventions are being tested or implemented – should consider questions such as: 1) Is the model of evaluation being used privileging certain kinds of interventions, organizations, and capacities? 2) Does building evidence about this particular intervention diminish investments in other, competing, interventions that remain untested? 3) Are you giving "bottom-up" solutions as much of a chance to demonstrate their efficacy as "top-down" solutions? 4) What are you doing to build capacity in community-based organizations serving unique populations or needs?

Potential loss of professional autonomy and leadership

A second concern regarding the future of human service organizations in the What Works era lies in how this approach might impact front-line staff and human service managers. Without a change in course, we foresee a reduced ability by the field of social work to provide professional leadership and expertise, as well as to articulate its own vision for promoting social welfare.

First, interventions that can be standardized and manualized are the more straightforward to evaluate and implement, and thus have florished in the EPB era. But assuming that any intervention can be truly "standardized" fles in the face of a long line of scholarship that has demonstrated that even when front-line staff are tasked with delivering uniform services, individual identity, preferences, judgments, and biases shape decision-making on the front lines. Michael Lipsky's classic, *Street-Level Bureaucracy* (Lipsky, 2010 [1980]) highlights the organizational constraints front-line workers endure, ultimately leading to disparate services and resources delivered to clients in the same programs. Other research has found that front-line workers will engage in tactics to bend (or sometimes break) program rules if they view program requirements as misaligned with client needs (Borry & Henderson, 2019; Brehm & Gates, 1999). More recent research has found that the racial and gender identities of front-line staff and clients interact in complex ways that might also differentially shape client experiences in social programs (Watkins-Hayes, 2009). Taken together, past scholarship on the heterogeneity of front-line practices in social programs should give researchers pause in assuming that tightly-designed caseworker-client interventions will not be susceptible to discretionary decision-making that may result in divergent "treatments" even within an evidence-based program.

Second, EBP's emphasis on standardized program models could lead to wide scale de-professionalization and undervaluing of front-line service providers in HSOs. If interaction with clients no longer requires training beyond implementing a specific protocol, why should organizations hire master's-level social workers, who are trained to, among other skills, serve clients by meeting them where they are? While some evidence-based techniques, like motivational interviewing, require workers to have designated levels of education or experience, highly manualized interventions do not rely on clinical judgment and in fact can discourage it in the name of "fidelity." Given the continuing financial pressure on HSOs, a perception that training on a particular intervention can substitute for general professional training may lead to fewer MSW-level positions. In addition, because EBPs require strict adherence to an intervention model, they also discourage workers from using their lived or professional experience in their practice. As HSOs (and social scientists) struggle to successfully replicate the effects of tested programs (Gamoran, 2018; Knox, Hill, & Berlin, 2018), especially with diverse client populations, front-line workers could offer a backstop. But this will only be true if skilled social workers and community leaders working in partnership are valued enough to still be employed on the front lines of HSOs.

The fate of social work-trained human service managers may be similar, yet different. HSOs already are becoming larger on average, with a greater proportion of the available funding being concentrated in a smaller number of organizations. As noted above, funding dynamics created by the demand for EBP place smaller organizations in jeopardy, further fueling the growth in average organizational size. These larger organizations create operational complexities that require more and different managerial skills, leading social workers to face increased competition for these jobs from other fields, including public administration, nonprofit management, and, in particular, business administration (Mirabella & Wish, 2000). This is occurring at a time when many schools of social work have anemic administrative tracks at best, and our graduates already are under-prepared to take the lead in increasingly complicated and professionalized HSOs.

These potential developments portend a future where social workers are required to treat every client using the same standardized intervention protocols, and are governed by a class of professionals who have not been trained in our field and may not share our professional values. As Mintzberg (2004) has noted, technocratic management is increasingly driving leaders with other "soft" skills out of leadership positions. If we believe that core social work values like equity, justice, and inclusion matter when working with marginalized populations, we should be concerned about this possible future. In management, particularly, it seems clear that there currently exists a mismatch between how we are preparing social workers in schools of social work and what is happening on the ground in HSOs. We thus face an important choice: either change what we are doing in social work education – i.e., train social work managers who can compete on skills regarding the use of evidence and advanced evaluation practices while holding on to social work values – or push back against what is happening in the field of HSOs. Most likely, the answer is to do some of both, but we need to engage these challenges now.

Neglect of the organizational context

Another reason to be concerned about the way the EBP movement is currently carried out is that it largely ignores the organizational context in which intervention models are implemented, and does little to foster organizational learning. Organizations are not just delivery platforms for interventions. Much as the social work "person-in-environment" perspective recognizes that individuals must be understood in the context of their family, community, and other relational settings, organizations are also situated in larger environments, and make decisions based on that context (Douglas, 1986). If human service managers resist implementing a program model "with fidelity," it is likely to be because one of the multiple, at times competing, external pressures faced by the organization is making it hard – even impossible – for "fidelity" to be assured (Meyer & Rowan, 1977; Weick, 1976). At times, the quest for "fidelity" may directly contradict a core commitment or relationship the organization holds, such as flexibility in client engagement. An understanding of these kinds of issues holds enormous power for determining whether and when program models will be successful at meeting their goals.

In fact, the tendency to move from intervention (often designed by an academic or other person not embedded in organizational context) to program deployment, without stopping to consider how the service delivery organization itself may affect the outcome means that many interventions may not be as successful as they might otherwise be. Enduring issues for implementation are the difficulty of changing organizational culture, the fact that new practices are initially a drain on performance as measured by benchmarks (requiring tolerance and patience by both managers and funders), and a lack of resources to fully implement the "active ingredients" in various change processes (Klein & Knight, 2005). Organizational norms and routines foster maintenance of the status quo, which often results in new interventions being at odds with existing organizational culture. Thus, without a good understanding of the existing organizational culture, external agents pushing for a change in organizational practices – e.g., academics, foundation leaders, consultants, and the like – are unlikely to convince organizational insiders that the new way is better.

Many scholars point to implementation science as a way of rectifying this problem. Implementation science promises to bridge the research-to-practice gap, showing how to encourage the adoption and improve the use of EBP (Aarons, Hurlburt, & Horwitz, 2011; Fisher, Shortell, & Savitz, 2016). This is important work and the field has been growing rapidly. Unfortunately, the way that most implementation science is currently done also often neglects the organizational dimension (Birken et al 2017). Implementation science is built on the assumption of top-down control – how to make an organization hew to what you want it to do – which aligns well with the need for program "fidelity" in organization-based evaluations. This is in stark contrast, however, to what organizational theorists would say about how best to achieve organizational change, as well as what the large body of literature on policy implementation has found regarding the success of such implementation efforts (Nilsen, Ståhl, Roback, & Cairney, 2013). In both fields, top-down efforts that are agnostic to organizational contexts are seen as likely to lead to dissent at the ground-level, ceremonial implementation, and long-term inefficiencies, not to mention reduced trust and staff morale.

There recently have been efforts to rectify the mismatch between organizational realities and the way that implementation science is practiced (e.g., Birken et al 2017; Jolles, Lengnick-Hall, & Mittman, 2019), but there is still a long way to go. Frameworks – like the Consolidated Framework for Implementation Research which includes contextual variation, adaptation, feedback, climate, and reflection (Damschroder et al. 2009) – exist that could point to new directions in partnering with organizations, but most research glosses over important contextual and learning dimensions.

Plus, implementation science is just one piece of the puzzle. Supporting effective implementation can only be done by leaders with a deep understanding of the organizational environment, skilled at resource generation and strategic administration, and knowledge of how to motivate and inspire the social work workforce (Sandfort & Moulton, 2014). We need greater scholarly attention – and funding to support research – regarding those things, too.

The organizational learning approach: a better way

Today's human service organizations increasingly find themselves confronting a high-stakes testing environment: show funders that your program model can produce experimental evidence of a causal effect, adopt one developed external to your organization, or risk losing critical financial support. As such, organizations' adoption of existing evidence-based models is often done as a fear response: a sure-fire path to poor implementation. What, then, might HSOs do instead? We argue that refocusing attention on organizational *learning* is required in order to truly build programs that work. This approach is also in alignment with a social work perspective. If we want research to be used to inform practice, we must do more to understand and promote the idea that the way research is used is always based on relationships, individual interpretation, and organizational realities, and will only be effectively done when organizations are open to learning, not held at knifepoint (Conaway, 2019).

An organizational learning approach rejects the idea that program fidelity is the only way to use evidence to inform human service delivery. This is because one of the clearest findings of the research on replication of EBP is that it is very difficult to expand or scale up the initial positive findings of a program model's causal effects. Indeed, articles in a 2018 special issue of the *Annals of the American Academy of Political and Social Sciences* on EBP repeatedly state that replication of evidence-based programming is the biggest problem faced by the field (e.g., Gamoran, 2018; Knox et al., 2018). Organizational learning instead favors an adaptive orientation to the use of evidence, such that the goal of program fidelity takes a back seat to systematically identifying program adaptations that will make service practices effective across a wider variety of populations, organizational contexts, and communities.

HSO managers are key actors in this process, and have long experimented with program innovations in response to new knowledge, new conditions, and new client populations (McBeath, Briggs, & Aisenberg, 2010). HSOs would benefit from researchers taking a more systematic approach to understanding how to equip managers with the skills necessary to play this role, as well as empowering managers to lead their teams in developing a learning orientation to their work. Organizational change is more likely to succeed when the diverse strengths of managers, front-line workers, and communities themselves are seen as assets, rather than potential impediments, to incorporating evidence for improved practice.

Practitioners can contribute to organizational learning by developing collaborative networks within which to share ideas, successes, and worries about different ways to use evidence to achieve better program outcomes. These relationships, built on professional trust and mutual investment over time, are key to shifting organizational practices so that research findings of various kinds can be incorporated into daily work (Conaway, 2019; Gamoran, 2018). This long-term, collaborative orientation to making research more useful to HSOs draws on longstanding findings about how organizational decisions are made: from an accumulation of information – including, but not limited to, research data – and a balancing of the different, sometimes competing demands faced by organizations. While policy mandates that tie organizational funding to the use of specific evidence-based practices may seek to sweep away this larger context of organizational decision-making, we believe such an approach will often find itself stymied by the complex realities of organizational life (Brown & Duguid, 1991).

One example of an organizational learning approach is the Breakthough Series Collaborative model, thus far used primarily in healthcare improvement (Kilo, 1998). This approach is based on building short-term (6–12 month) multi-level learning communities where participants share experiences while undertaking similar kinds of organizational change (such as implementing a new evidence-based approach). Built on capturing the benefits of dialog over didactic settings when working with professionals, it respects the hard-won knowledge of those on the front lines, allows for flexibility in implementation, and promotes mutual learning. This type of approach is an investment, but such approaches will allow us to reinvest in community-based organizations and advance the knowledge that they have while also building their capacity.

Implications

In order to envision a future for human service organizations and management that is focused on promoting social change and equity as well as professional autonomy and respect, we advocate adopting such an organizational learning perspective. We also suggest three further adjustments to social work research trends in order to refocus our attention toward research that is more colla-borative with affected communities, attentive to the self-determination of consumers, and targeted more toward the reform of economic and societal structures. These suggestions, as well as others discussed above, are summarized in Table 1.

Table 1. Research strategies to advance equity in the "What works" movement and promote organizational learning.

Challenge	Suggested Research Strategies
Support community-based knowledge	• Develop strategies for smaller, community-based organizations to appro-priately evaluate their practices • Give "bottom-up" programming the same chance to demonstrate efficacy as "top-down" programming
Protect autonomy and professional leadership in the social work workforce	• Determine the diversity of skills (technical and relational) managers need to excel in leading human service organizations • Assess how existing practitioner knowledge can be better integrated with evidence-based protocols on the ground
Foreground the organizational and community context	• Determine the ways in which context interacts with outcomes in EBP interventions • Investigate the replicability of effective adaptations
Improve the contextual implementation of EBPs	• Observe front-line staff and client interactions to reveal both promises and challenges of new service delivery practices that might be overlooked by relying solely on outcome assessments • Leverage worker knowledge to build better implementation protocols
Facilitate organizational learning *across* agencies	• Compare agencies with different client groups to assess how EBPs are being implemented, and the impact on organizational functioning and client outcomes • Implement collaborative learning groups across organizations in similar practice domains to share promising adaptations
Facilitate organizational learning *within* agencies	• Assess the use of learning groups comprised of staff at various levels of the organization in order to enhance communication, EBP adaptation, and manager and front-line staff trust and communication • Engage in rapid assessment of practices so organizations can learn as they implement and adapt EBPs
Ensure research promotes meaningful and equitable social change	• Focus attention on agency practices and EBPs that promote structural change as much as behavioral change • Work to make visible the aspects of social work and agency practice not accounted for in traditional program metrics

First, a key part of the social work tradition is our emphasis on seeing how inequality at the macro level of policies and communities can lead to wildly divergent outcomes at the micro level of individuals and families. This should be a strength of the profession at the present moment when awareness about the enduring effects of racism, educational inequality, and disinvestment in poor communities is at an all-time high. The rise of politicians like Stacey Abrams, Alexandria Ocasio-Cortez, and Bernie Sanders can be traced to the ways they are calling out how current U.S. health care, tax, and labor policies create inequality on the ground, benefiting the rich at the expense of the poor, usually in ways that are also racially coded. It is ironic, then, that at this moment, social work is instead investing in interventions that place the onus of responsibility for change on the affected individual.

As an example of what we mean, consider this incomplete list of ways we could address the problem of income inequality: minimum wage increases, baby bonds, reparations for chattel slavery, expanded labor rights, tax reform, and minimum income guarantees. All of these solutions place responsibility for the issue within economic and political systems. But the kind of interventions that are typically being tested and promoted by social workers are based on changing the activities and behaviors of the poor: asset development programs, mentoring programs, college readiness programs, and the like. These programs are important, and may change the lives of those who participate in them, but they ultimately will not, nor are they designed to, transform societal structures or effect sweeping economic and political change. We argue that because the EBP movement is not well-suited to addressing the structural causes of inequality, it is – unintentionally – causing the profession to focus its intellectual attention away from social reform work. Our scholarship and advocacy should be directed toward improving the quality or number of jobs that currently exist and ensuring greater equity in employment and compensation, *as well as* designing better job training programs and procuring funding for them.

Second, we also call for increased attention to the potential impact on the communities most likely to be subjected to "neutral" scientific approaches. These often comprise people from historically marginalized groups – such as those who are poor, disabled, formerly incarcerated, immigrants, Black and Brown, or gender non-conforming. While we do not claim that offering services to marginalized communities through interventions under evaluation is in itself a bad thing, it does mean that these communities are disproportionately subjected to the "behavior changing" interventions described above. This may reaffirm the view that people on the margins simply need to be "fixed," thereby situating the problem within the individual or family. Given the proliferation of behavioral change research in our profession, this is more evidence of how the social work gaze has unwittingly shifted away from more macro-level interventions, such as broad economic security policies. This shift in focus harkens back to previous tensions in the field between social change versus medicalized practice that was believed to foster professionalization (Specht & Courtney, 1994). At this juncture of the rise of EBP, we still have time to interrogate the meaning and implications of such approaches for those we are most bound to serve through our values of social, racial, and economic justice.

Finally, we need to recognize the relational nature of our work and that perhaps "program fidelity" should not be a more important goal than social service delivery that is personalized, respects self-determination, collaborates with marginalized communities, and is tailored to community needs. Social work managers and front-line staff have strengths in interpersonal skills, coming from their clinical training and the general orientation to human dignity that is a core value of the field. Indeed, it is the way our profession centers the individual, family, and community in our scholarship, advocacy, and day-to-day work that renders it uniquely qualified to comment on and respond to the implications of "neutral" science and methods.

How might social work researchers incorporate these concerns into their work? In the broadest sense, it means developing a better understanding of how multiple forms of knowledge and evidence – not just experimental "gold standard" evidence – can contribute to effective social work practice. For example, research on "relational work" (Benjamin & Campbell 2015) demonstrates the many ways that HSOs and social workers assist clients that are not accounted for in traditional program metrics, and thus rendered essentially invisible. What are the other aspects of HSO work that are similarly unrecognized, and how might they be made more visible? Another important question is the one that was posed a decade ago by McBeath et al. (2010): Do we have a strong basis for believing that EBPs actually provide promised benefits to a wide range of clients and communities? Their systematic review of the evidence argued that we do not; together with the recent work lamenting the lack of EBP replicability, it seems time for a new assessment of the evidence to date. Now that federal and state governments increasingly are mandating that HSOs use EBPs to obtain public funds, we need empirical examination more than ever of what the effects of such mandates are on clients, communities, and HSOs themselves. We worry that the push for HSOs to "adopt" and "implement" evidence instead of learning from and adapting it may further marginalize vulnerable communities and the profession more generally. Instead, we, along with the communities we serve, must stake our claim on improving evaluative efforts that better account for organizational reality as well as community values and needs.

Disclosure statement

No potential conflict of interest was reported by the authors.

ORCID

Jennifer E. Mosley ⓘ http://orcid.org/0000-0002-9292-6710

References

Aarons, G. A., Hurlburt, M., & Horwitz, S. M. (2011). Advancing a conceptual model of evidence-based practice implementation in public service sectors. *Administration and Policy in Mental Health and Mental Health Services Research*, 38(1), 4–23. doi:10.1007/s10488-010-0327-7

Abbott, A. (1995). Boundaries of social work or social work of boundaries? *Social Service Review*, 69, 545–562. doi:10.1086/604148

Benjamin, L. M., & Campbell, D. C. (2015). Nonprofit performance: accounting for the agency of clients. *Nonprofit and Voluntary Sector Quarterly*, 44(5), 988–1006. doi:10.1177/0899764014551987

Birken, S. A., Bunger, A. C., Powell, B. J., Turner, K., Clary, A. S., Klaman, S. L., ... Rostad, W. L. (2017). Organizational theory for dissemination and implementation research. *Implementation Science*, 12(1), 62. doi:10.1186/s13012-017-0592-x

Boris, E. T., de Leon, E., Roeger, K., & Nikolova, M. (2010). *Human service nonprofits and government collaboration: Findings from the 2010 national survey of nonprofit government contracting and grants*. Washington, DC: Urban Institute.

Borry, E. L., & Henderson, A. C. (2019). Patients, protocols, and prosocial behavior: Rule breaking in Frontline Health Care. *The American Review of Public Administration*, 0275074019862680. https://doi.org/10.1177/027507401-9862680

Bouris, A., Voisin, D., Pilloton, M., Flatt, N., Eavou, R., Hampton, K., ... Schneider, J. A. (2013). Project nGage: Network supported HIV care engagement for younger black men who have sex with men and transgender persons. *Journal of AIDS & Clinical Research*, 4(9), 236.

Brehm, J. O., & Gates, S. (1999). *Working, shirking, and sabotage: Bureaucratic response to a democratic public*. Ann Arbor, MI: University of Michigan Press.

Brown, J. S., & Duguid, P. (1991). Organizational learning and communities-of-practice: Toward a unified view of working, learning, and innovation. *Organization Science*, 2(1), 40–57. doi:10.1287/orsc.2.1.40

Carman, J. G., & Fredericks, K. A. (2008). Nonprofits and evaluation: empirical evidence from the field. *New Directions for Evaluation*, 2008(119), 51–71.

Conaway, C. 2019. *Maximizing research use in the world we actually live In: Relationships, organizations, and interpretation*. CALDER Policy Brief No. 14-0319-1. (CALDER Opinion Brief). Washington, D.C.: National Center for Analysis of Longitudinal Data in Education Research.

Damschroder, L. J., Aron, D. C., Keith, R. E., Kirsh, S. R., Alexander, J. A., & Lowery, J. C. (2009). Fostering implementation of health services research findings into practice: a consolidated framework for advancing implementation science. *Implementation Science*, 4(1), 50. doi:10.1186/1748-5908-4-50

Deegan, M. J. (1988). *Jane Addams and the men of the Chicago School, 1892–1918*. Chicago, IL: University of Chicago Press.

Douglas, M. (1986). *How institutions think*. Syracuse, NY: Syracuse University Press.

Fisher, E. S., Shortell, S. M., & Savitz, L. A. (2016). Implementation science: A potential catalyst for delivery system reform. *JAMA, 315*(4), 339–340. doi:10.1001/jama.2015.17949

Gamoran, A. (2018). Evidence-based policy in the real world: A cautionary view. *Annals of the American Academy of Political and Social Sciences, 678*, 180–191. doi:10.1177/0002716218770138

Green, K. R. 2018. Exploring the implications of shifting HIV prevention practice ideologies on the work of community-based organizations: A resource dependence perspective. Unpublished Ph.D. Dissertation, University of Chicago.

Hurdle, D. E. (2002). Native Hawaiian traditional healing: Culturally based interventions for social work practice. *Social Work, 47*(2), 183–192.

Jolles, M. P., Lengnick-Hall, R., & Mittman, B. S. (2019). Core functions and forms of complex health interventions: A patient-centered medical home illustration. *Journal of General Internal Medicine*. doi:10.1007/s11606-019-04885-z

Kilo, C. M. (1998). A framework for collaborative improvement: Lessons from the Institute for healthcare improvement's breakthrough series. *Quality Management in Health Care, 6*(4), 1–13.

Klein, K. J., & Knight, A. P. (2005). Innovation Implementation: Overcoming the challenge. *Current Directions in Psychological Science, 14*, 243–246. doi:10.1111/j.0963-7214.2005.00373.x

Knox, V., Hill, C. J., & Berlin, G. (2018). Can evidence-based policy ameliorate the nation's social problems? *Annals of the American Academy of Political and Social Sciences, 678*, 166–179. doi:10.1177/0002716218769844

Lipsky, M. (2010 [1980]). *Street-level bureaucracy: Dilemmas of the individual in public service*. New York, NY: Russell Sage Foundation.

McBeath, B., Briggs, H. E., & Aisenberg, E. (2010). Examining the premises supporting the empirically supported intervention approach to social work practice. *Social Work, 55*(4), 347–357.

Meyer, J. W., & Rowan, B. (1977). Institutionalized Organizations: Formal structure as myth and ceremony. *American Journal of Sociology, 83*(2), 340–363. doi:10.1086/226550

Mintzberg, H. (2004). *Managers, not MBAs: A hard look at the soft practice of managing and management development*. San Francisco, CA: Berrett-Koehler Publishers.

Mirabella, R. M., & Wish, N. B. (2000). The "Best place" Debate: A comparison of graduate education programs for nonprofit managers. *Public Administration Review, 60*, 219–229. doi:10.1111/0033-3352.00082

Nilsen, P., Ståhl, C., Roback, K., & Cairney, P. (2013). Never the Twain shall meet? A comparison of implementation science and policy implementation research. *Implementation Science, 8*(1), 63. doi:10.1186/1748-5908-8-63

Salamon, L. M. (1995). *Partners in public service: Government-nonprofit relations in the modern welfare state*. Baltimore, MD: Johns Hopkins University Press.

Sandfort, J., & Moulton, S. (2014). *Effective implementation in practice: Integrating public policy and management*. Hoboken, NJ: John Wiley & Sons.

Satterfield, J. M., Spring, B., Brownson, R. C., Mullen, E. J., Newhouse, R. P., Walker, B. B., & Whitlock, E. P. (2009). Toward a transdisciplinary model of evidence-based practice. *Milbank Quarterly, 87*(2), 368–390. doi:10.1111/j.1468-0009.2009.00561.x

Specht, H., & Courtney, M. E. (1994). *Unfaithful angels: How social work has abandoned its mission*. New York, NY: Free Press.

Spencer, M. S., Rosland, A.-M., Kieffer, E. C., Sinco, B. R., Valerio, M., Palmisano, G., ... Heisler, M. (2011). Effectiveness of a community health worker intervention among African American and Latino adults with type 2 diabetes: A randomized controlled trial. *American Journal of Public Health, 101*(12), 2253–2260. doi:10.2105/AJPH.2010.300106

Stivers, C. (2000). *Bureau men, settlement women: Constructing public administration in the progressive era*. Lawrence, KS: University Press of Kansas.

Watkins-Hayes, C. (2009). *The new welfare bureaucrats: Entanglements of race, class, and policy reform*. Chicago, IL: University of Chicago Press.

Weick, K. E. (1976). Educational organizations as loosely coupled systems. *Administrative Science Quarterly, 21*, 1–19. doi:10.2307/2391875

De-Implementation of Evidence-Based Interventions: Implications for Organizational and Managerial Research

Rogério M. Pinto and Sunggeun (Ethan) Park

ABSTRACT

The science of implementing evidence-based interventions (EBIs) is being developed in social work and many other disciplines. Particular attention has been paid to whether, when, and how to de-implement an EBI if that intervention turns out to be harmful and/or a more effective/efficient EBI becomes available. Current research focuses on investigating how various environmental-, organizational-, provider-, and client-level factors influence the de-implementation process. Grounded in the HIV prevention field of inquiry and organizational theories, herein, we explore several issues that influence implementation and de-implementation and share key points for further investigation. Recommendations for future research are also discussed.

Introduction

Social work's interest in evidence-based practices has contributed to the growing attention to implementation research – the "study of processes and strategies that move, or integrate, evidence-based effective treatments into routine use, in usual care settings" (Proctor et al., 2009, p. 27). Implementation research stems from the recognition that, despite the significant advancements in understanding the causes of biopsychosocial problems and the subsequent development of innovations to address them, biomedical and behavioral health research have made little impact on the quality or effectiveness of health services – particularly due to the research-to-practice gap (Institute of Medicine, 2001). Studies show that newly developed evidence-based practices may take, on average, between 15 and 20 years to be incorporated into routine practices (Bauer, Damschroder, Hagedorn, Smith, & Kilbourne, 2015; Proctor et al., 2009). Delays in implementation have resulted in patients receiving delayed recommended prevention and care; for example, 55% of diabetic patients, 63% of patients with sexually transmitted diseases, and 89% of patients suffering from alcohol use disorder, to name just a few areas (McGlynn et al., 2003). The implementation science literature emerged to address both the need for testing intervention effectiveness in diverse care environments (beyond efficacy within a tightly controlled setting), and for improving uptake and implementation of interventions deemed to be effective.

For the past few decades, researchers advanced knowledge on how various factors at multiple levels (e.g., environment-, organization-, provider-, and user-levels) may influence evidence-based intervention implementation, how intervention adoption may impact organizational practices and behaviors, and how some human, social, and public health service organizations may adopt interventions more successfully than others (Palinkas & Soydan, 2012). However, for the past recent years, implementation research has added a significant focus toward de-implementation – "the discontinuation of interventions that should no longer be provided" (McKay, Morshed, Brownson,

This article has been republished with minor change. This change do not impact the academic content of the article.
Color versions of one or more of the figures in the article can be found online at www.tandfonline.com/wasw.

Proctor, & Prusaczyk, 2018, p. 190). Decades of implementation research have accumulated evidence about intervention impact, and best practices regarding uptake and delivery. Based on this evidence, funders have prioritized the support of more cost-effective interventions. This new focus has prompted a call for research aimed at interrogating when and how it might be appropriate to de-emphasize and, ultimately, stop delivering interventions when an existing intervention (1) turns out to be harmful, and/or (2) when a more efficient or effective intervention becomes available (Brownson et al., 2015; National Institutes of Health, 2009; Niven et al., 2015; Ogden & Fixsen, 2014). Analogous to the implementation process, de-implementation can be influenced by environmental (e.g., changes in regulations and resource flows), organizational (e.g., capacity for staff training and history of organizational change), and both provider- and client-level factors (e.g., provider's experience and client's preferences). Recent research has begun to show that de-implementation may also be influenced by time-sensitive variables, such as new policies and regulations (for example, see Pinto, Witte, Filippone, Choi, & Wall, 2018b).

De-implementation is a critical issue that human service organization researchers, policy-makers, and managers will need to evaluate now and in the foreseeable future. Given many human service fields' growing emphasis on evidence-based practices and increasing evidence on existing programs' effectiveness, the cost-effective approach is spreading rapidly across the health and social service fields. For instance, in the child welfare service field, under the Family First Prevention Services Act of 2018, new federal funding will be only available for programs reviewed and approved by the California Evidence-Based Clearinghouse on Child Welfare (National Conference of State Legislatures, 2019). In the homelessness service field, the U.S. Department of Housing and Urban Development, perhaps the most important provider of funding in this field, recognized a Housing First approach as a cost-effective intervention over other approaches and prioritized regional service networks offering permanent supportive housing for the chronically homeless (U.S. Department of Housing and Urban Development, 2014).

Herein, we begin a discussion about our efforts aimed at understanding relationships between implementation and de-implementation processes and how de-implementation may have an impact on newly emphasized practices. Specifically, we focus on the behaviors of social and public health service providers in the field of HIV prevention as a case in point. We address de-implementation of interventions of a long-running program, the Centers for Disease Control and Prevention's (CDC) Diffusion of Effective [HIV Prevention] Behavioral Interventions (DEBI). We explore how long-running behavioral interventions, now being de-implemented, may influence the implementation of new types of interventions (e.g., biomedical). This paper shows how new interventions may contribute to shaping the behaviors of service providers in the HIV prevention field while highlighting issues of importance for other human service fields. Implications and recommendations for implementation and de-implementation studies and practices will follow.

Background: shift in evidence-based HIV prevention interventions

In the early 2010s, the CDC began to de-emphasize and de-implement most evidence-based HIV prevention interventions (HIV EBIs) that had been widely adopted for more than 20 years. The CDC has called for a more effective and efficient High-Impact HIV Prevention approach (i.e., increased referrals to biobehavioral services for high-risk groups) that requires intense interagency and interprofessional collaborations (Centers for Disease Control and Prevention, 2017). During 2011–2012, the CDC launched the High-Impact HIV Prevention approach to integrate high-impact and efficient interventions in geographically defined diffusion systems across the country targeting groups most vulnerable to HIV infection, such as men who have sex with men, communities of color, women, injection drug users, and transgender women (CDC, 2011).

The shift in the CDC's priority and focus triggered changes in how organization managers and service providers operate and serve high-risk clients in the United States and around the globe. Under the new approach, the CDC halted their financial support of nearly half of the HIV EBIs that had been widely promoted for more than two decades, unless they are currently deemed to be cost-effective for targeted populations with significant HIV burdens (CDC, 2017). The High-Impact HIV Prevention approach requires providers to: (1) refer high-risk individuals of unknown HIV status to be tested for HIV, and (2) make referrals to HIV primary care, to biobehavioral interventions [e.g., STIs, Hepatitis-C testing and treatment, and pre-exposure prophylaxis (PrEP)], to support services (e.g., drug treatment and mental health), and to structural interventions (e.g., syringe exchange programs). Because many HIV prevention programs do not offer such a wide array of services, the newly promoted High-Impact HIV Prevention approach requires intense collaborations across service organizations and service providers with a renewed focus on HIV prevention. This shift in HIV prevention priorities provides a timely opportunity to understand better a key question: How exposure to de-implemented interventions (i.e., CDC EBIs) may influence the implementation of interventions currently emphasized by the CDC (i.e., High-Impact HIV Prevention approach)?

Conceptual foundation

In order to explore this question, we propose a conceptual model that depicts interactive and dynamic relationships between the evolution of the CDC's HIV intervention strategies and various factors with the potential to influence implementation. Implementation models stress internal, external, and network-based factors that may influence different implementation phases – exploration, preparation/adoption, active implementation, and sustainment. These models are based on multiple theories, and they describe policies, and individual, client, provider, and organization factors affecting implementation behaviors (Aarons, Hurlburt, & Horwitz, 2011; Birken et al., 2017). Reflecting implementation models, we suggest a framework depicting factors at different levels shaping the transition between CDC EBIs and High-Impact Prevention. Our framework integrates principles from select theoretical viewpoints in order to describe organizational adaptive behavior to new conditions over some time. Herein, we focus on select factors at several levels, and not on identifying temporal processes of organizational change (e.g., critical events or stages of organizational change) – such an endeavor would require substantial discussions regarding each cycle and event, and this is outside the scope of this paper (Kaufmann, 1993; Mohr, 1982).

Figure 1 depicts environmental, organizational, and provider-level factors linked by vertical arrows representing their inter-connectedness. The new institutional theory suggests that CDC's emphasis on the implementation of EBIs up until the 2000s imposed multiple pressures, especially through altering funding support policy (i.e., regulatory pressure) and emphasizing the cost-

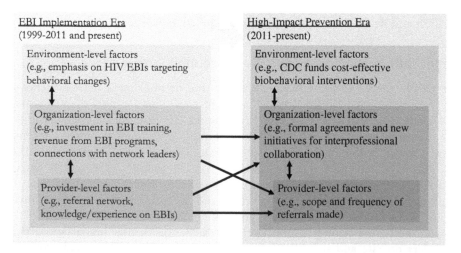

Figure 1. Factors influencing implementation/(de)implementation in a time of transition and beyond.

effectiveness of a new approach (i.e., normative pressure) (DiMaggio & Powell, 1983). To reduce uncertainty and secure financial and political resources, HIV prevention service organizations had to make a strategic decision to optimize organizational structures, procedures, and outputs for EBI delivery (Oliver, 1991; Pfeffer & Salancik, 1978). To improve the organizational fit to its operating environment, many organizations might have offered training opportunities for their staff to provide multiple EBIs that can bring in more revenue to their organizations (Ruef, 2000; Veniegas, Kao, Rosales, & Arellanes, 2009). Under new mandates, many providers were exposed to EBIs not just through formal training but also through discussing the strengths and weaknesses of EBIs with colleagues – as the social network theory would suggest (Burt, 1992). Both formally and informally, providers developed referral networks to address unmet health and social service needs of clients.

The systems theory suggests that environmental, organizational, and provider-level factors, in the period promoting HIV EBIs, could have influenced how HIV prevention service organizations and providers experienced and adapted to the new era promoting High-Impact HIV Prevention services (represented with horizontal and diagonal arrows in Figure 1). For example, compared to organizations that relied more heavily on the CDC's funding, organizations serving more privately insured clients (particularly those who may prefer to continue to receive EBIs) may strategically delay their adoption of the new approach or continue to offer some EBIs (Oliver, 1991; Pfeffer & Salancik, 1978). Organizations might transition to the High-Impact HIV Prevention approach more easily if their managers are well connected with systems leaders (e.g., public administrators or private foundation program officers) during the EBI implementation era. Leveraging their networks, these organizations can learn about the upcoming changes in the field (e.g., funders' priorities and preferences for resource allocation) and be better prepared and positioned for the new approach (Gifford, Graham, Ehrhart, Davies, & Aarons, 2017; Palinkas et al., 2011). Providers developed transferable skills through offering EBIs as they also developed strong networks for referral-making, and thus prepared the way for integrating high-impact interventions and for referring clients to myriad different providers of social and biobehavioral services (Dolcini et al., 2010). When more providers within an organization find an external organization as a trustworthy partner, the organization may initiate a formal agreement for referrals that can reduce the cost in searching for collaboration partners as the transaction cost theory suggests (Coase, 1988).

Exposure to CDC EBIs influences the implementation of high-impact HIV prevention

Grounded in the theories explored above, we conducted a study that involved 379 HIV service providers. The study aimed to examine the implementation of myriad HIV prevention services across 36 agencies in New York City. Figure 1 above provides a depiction of the temporal connection between the EBI Implementation Era and the High-Impact Prevention (HIP) Era, a staged social work public health approach to prevention. The EBI Era (1999–2011 and present) was followed by the HIP Era (2011–present) which now includes *all* high impact services. The EBI Era is hypothesized to influence provider behaviors in the HIP Era, such as referral-making. Here, we focus specifically on how exposure to EBIs may influence the rate at which providers make linkages to high impact services.

Our research shows significant associations between provider's exposure to the CDC's evidence-based interventions and the frequency at which they made referrals to different high-impact, newly emphasized services (Pinto, Witte, Filippone, Choi, & Wall, 2018a) as follows. Providers exposed to *any* CDC EBI more frequently referred clients to HIV, HEP-C, and STI testing, to primary care, drug treatment, and mental health services. Furthermore, exposure to more than one CDC EBI resulted in more frequent referrals to these services. Exposure was conceptualized based on whether social and public health service providers worked for organizations that were funded to provide CDC EBIs. The study concluded that exposure to many of the CDC's EBIs, although they are now de-implemented, may have contributed to the relative success of newly implemented biobehavioral interventions.

Using the same data from the study described above, we examined whether provider perceptions on interprofessional collaboration were associated with their referral-making behaviors. The study found that providers who regarded interprofessional collaboration positively make more referrals to HIV testing and primary care every week (Pinto et al., 2018a). However, de-implementation may introduce unwelcome impacts on interprofessional collaboration that could shape the provider's referral practice. For example, one study shows that de-implementation of RESPECT, a CDC EBI, has weakened relationships with interagency collaboration partners (McKay et al., 2018). The evidence from our qualitative study also demonstrated that, despite growing expectations for interagency and interprofessional collaboration, providers are often reluctant to make referrals to other agencies for fear of losing clients, particularly to those organizations which do not engage in *mutual* referral-making (Pinto et al., 2018b).

De-implementation of the CDC's EBIs might also have influenced agency environments (e.g., diminished revenue from behavioral interventions, downsizing of staff and physical space, and lack of technical resources and assistance) all of which may have produced a negative impact on referral-making (Gandelman, DeSantis, & Rietmeijer, 2006). In sum, de-implementation of an intervention may deter or delay successful implementation of a new approach through various mechanisms, such as the disruption of existing relationships and demanding organizational change and adjustment to a new environment.

Implications and recommendations

Research on de-implementation has just begun. Our overall recommendation for researchers developing evidence-based interventions is that they study in more detail all stages of implementation – including adoption, sustainability, and exit – before developing and testing new interventions. Implementations require training providers to deliver new and different programs, but it also incurs dynamic changes – practices, organizational structures, and possibly environmental contexts – that can linger after an implementation or de-implementation process. Thus, thinking through the impact that a new intervention will bring into different phases of implementation will illuminate de-implementation research, especially in terms of how less effective and possibly harmful approaches can be de-implemented in a more timely, systematic, and safe manner.

Moving forward, implementation research with a focus on organization and management will benefit from exploring the many actors involved in the decision-making process concerning de-implementation of well-known and previously adopted interventions vis-à-vis their replacement by less-known and, often, less popular HIV-prevention practices. The extant literature on implementation has mainly focused on the adoption-implementation-sustainment process, but it has neglected political, institutional, organizational and cultural factors that help to drive the replacement of interventions in the HIV-prevention and other fields of practice. One major issue, which deserves current and future attention, concerns community exclusion from decision-making processes related to intervention implementation. The inclusion of community members and practitioners (deliverers of interventions) in implementation research and practice may improve our understanding of ecological factors influencing, directly and indirectly, the implementation of myriad practices in different fields of interest (Pinto & Witte, 2019).

There is great potential for organizational and management scholars to improve our understanding on how human, social, and public health service organizations and providers behave and navigate the transition between de-implementation of an intervention and implementation of new ones. Research is sorely needed on how specific factors may influence the implementation of new interventions with a focus on the context (i.e., regional competition and existing referral networks) in which administrators and providers make decisions regarding de-implementation processes. Qualitative studies on how directors wrestle with de-implementation and implementation decisions and strategically navigate pressures to offer cost-effective programs over responsive services could yield more practical suggestions for organizational management. For instance, directors of organizations providing evidence-based programs adapted to racial/ethnic minority groups may be reluctant to abandon previous programs. They may rather take strategic approaches, such as offering both previous and newly emphasized programs while advocating the importance of culturally sensitive interventions.

We contend that it is also critical that researchers develop more research to describe the replacement process; in other words, what happens after an intervention is de-implemented? For example, research is needed in order to understand better instances in which HIV providers may de-implement an intervention in response to policy and practice changes, but not necessarily offer a new intervention – "a replacement." This is an area in great need of attention by organizational scholars to understand empirically the nuances of de-implementation and replacement practices in an institutional environment. Longitudinal research is particularly recommended for this purpose.

Concurrently, more attention will be needed in advancing theories and developing methods that could more specifically guide research on organizational-level variables (e.g., professionalization, revenue sources, internal policies, staff and client compositions, etcetera) as key factors that may influence de-implementation practices as well as policy. Beyond widely used theories in the implementation literature (e.g., theories on innovation diffusion, social network, leadership, systems, and organizational adaptation and learning), scholars are encouraged to refine traditional theories and bring together new perspectives to frame the implementation and de-implementation phenomena and their implications. Better targeted public support for implementation can be derived from exploring what incentivizes providers to adopt new practices, despite their situation in-between escalating demands and limited resources, using the street-level bureaucracy theory (Brodkin, 2011; Lipsky, 1980). How client's direct and indirect representation in de-implementation and implementation processes is another promising area of research particularly for social work scholars, given client's expertise from lived experience and their limited opportunities to influence service decisions in many human, social, and public health service settings (Meier, 1993; Park, 2019).

In terms of methods, we encourage researchers to pay more attention to community perceptions on the de-implementation and implementation processes. Researchers often fail to include clients and providers as partners in the design, testing, and dissemination of interventions. This oversight and partnership may have dire implications in designing interventions, implementing and de-implementing interventions, and examining and improving processes. For example, clients who are most vulnerable to HIV acquisition often reject the implementation of services that may be too hard to access, too long to deliver, whose effect is not immediate, or services that are not culturally competent. Given the history of abuses by researchers (e.g., Tuskegee syphilis study), clients, providers, and also agency administrators are known to be suspicious of research evidence and to reject research products. Invested and trusted community partnerships will allow researchers to have difficult but imperative discussions on 'what did not work' and how to improve intervention designs and better support implementation/de-implementation processes. The end-product of this participatory process would be more relevant and could potentially generate responsive interventions and approaches that can be implemented as designed and de-implemented with limited footmarks. Therefore, meaningful inclusion of community members (including managers, providers, and clients) is of paramount importance, particularly for de-implementation and implementation research.

We end this perspective paper with a cautionary comment. Growing interests in implementation and de-implementation research offer both opportunities and risks to the organizational scholarship within the field of social work and beyond. Organizational and contextual dimensions of human, social, and health service production have been understudied, and a focus toward implementation and de-implementation offers great potential for advancing knowledge on the impacts of environmental pressures and demands, organizational structures and constraints, staff characteristics and capacities, and client's roles to name a few. At the same time, unbalanced attention toward one area of organizational scholarship is a concerning trend. Human service organizations have been considered as venues for not just health and social service provision, but civic engagement, empowerment, community organizing, and social change (Hasenfeld & Garrow, 2012; Park, Mosley, & Grogan, 2016). Organizational studies simply facilitating and fueling service implementation and de-implementation can harm the overall missions of the social work profession and scholarship. Many scholars and practitioners have legitimate concerns on pervasive emphases on the evidence-based practices across the field of social work that can de-legitimatize bottom-up community-based learning, de-value professional service providers' expertise and autonomy, and privilege particular types of interventions and organizations (see Mosley, Marwell, and Ybarra's (2019) commentary in this issue). Thus, for maintaining and further developing organizational and management scholarship that can contribute to social work's overall mission of distributive justice restoration for the disadvantaged and marginalized, even-handed investment and attention are needed in imperative research domains, including but not limited to how staff and user's expertise can improve implementation and de-implementation processes, whether and how human service organization managers resist pressures to use cost-effective interventions over responsive and relevant services for communities they serve, and how service providers and users can lead institutional change.

Disclosure statement

No potential conflict of interest was reported by the authors.

References

Aarons, G. A., Hurlburt, M., & Horwitz, S. M. (2011). Advancing a conceptual model of evidence-based practice implementation in public service sectors. *Administration and Policy in Mental Health*, 38(1), 4–23. doi:10.1007/s10488-010-0327-7

Bauer, M. S., Damschroder, L., Hagedorn, H., Smith, J., & Kilbourne, A. M. (2015). An introduction to implementation science for the non-specialist. *BMC Psychology*, 3, 1. doi:10.1186/s40359-015-0089-9

Birken, S. A., Bunger, A. C., Powell, B. J., Turner, K., Clary, A. S., Klaman, S. L., ... Weiner, B. J. (2017). Organizational theory for dissemination and implementation research. *Implementation Science*, 12(1), 62. doi:10.1186/s13012-017-0592-x

Brodkin, E. Z. (2011). Policy work: Street-level organizations under new managerialism. *Journal of Public Administration Research and Theory*, 21(2), i253–i277. doi:10.1093/jopart/muq093

Brownson, R. C., Allen, P., Jacob, R. R., Harris, J. K., Duggan, K., Hipp, P. R., & Erwin, P. C. (2015). Understanding mis-implementation in public health practice. *American Journal of Preventive Medicine*, 48(5), 543–551. doi:10.1016/j.amepre.2014.11.015

Burt, R. S. (1992). *Structural holes: The social structure of competition*. Cambridge, MA: Harvard University Press.

Centers for Disease Control and Prevention. (2011). *High-impact HIV prevention: CDC's approach to reducing HIV infections in the United States*. Centers for Disease Control and Prevention National Center for HIV/AIDS, Viral Hepatitis, STD, and TB Prevention Division of HIV/AIDS Prevention. Retrieved from https://www.cdc.gov/hiv/pdf/policies_nhpc_booklet.pdf

Centers for Disease Control and Prevention. (2017). *High impact HIV Prevention (HIP): Overview of select interventions & strategies*. Washington, DC: Danya International.

Coase, R. H. (1988). The nature of the firm: Influence. *The Journal of Law, Economics, and Organization*, 4(1), 33–47. doi:10.1093/oxfordjournals.jleo.a036947

DiMaggio, P. J., & Powell, W. W. (1983). The iron cage revisited: Institutional isomorphism and collective rationality in organizational fields. *American Sociological Review*, 48(2), 147–160. doi:10.2307/2095101

Dolcini, M. M., Gandelman, A., Vogan, S. A., Kong, C., Leak, T.-N., King, A. J., ... O'Leary, A. (2010). Translating HIV interventions into practice: Community-based organizations' experiences with the Diffusion of Effective Behavioral Interventions (DEBIs). *Social Science & Medicine (1982)*, 71(10), 1839–1846. doi:10.1016/j.socscimed.2010.08.011

Gandelman, A. A., DeSantis, L. M., & Rietmeijer, C. A. (2006). Assessing community needs and agency capacity—An integral part of implementing effective evidence–Based interventions. *AIDS Education and Prevention*, 18(supp), 32–43. doi:10.1521/aeap.2006.18.supp.32

Gifford, W., Graham, I. D., Ehrhart, M. G., Davies, B. L., & Aarons, G. A. (2017, March 29). Ottawa model of implementation leadership and implementation leadership scale: Mapping concepts for developing and evaluating theory-based leadership interventions. *Journal of Healthcare Leadership*. doi:10.2147/JHL.S125558

Hasenfeld, Y., & Garrow, E. E. (2012). Nonprofit human-service organizations, social rights, and advocacy in a neoliberal welfare State. *Social Service Review*, 86(2), 295–322. doi:10.1086/666391

Institute of Medicine. (2001). *Crossing the quality chasm: A new health system for the 21st century*. USA: National Academies Press. Retrieved from https://www.ncbi.nlm.nih.gov/books/NBK222274/

Kaufmann, S. (1993). *The origins of order*. New York, NY: Oxford University Press.

Lipsky, M. (1980). *Street-level bureaucracy: Dilemmas of the individual in public services.* New York, NY: Russell Sage Foundation.

McGlynn, E. A., Asch, S. M., Adams, J., Keesey, J., Hicks, J., DeCristofaro, A., & Kerr, E. A. (2003). The quality of health care delivered to adults in the United States. *New England Journal of Medicine, 348*(26), 2635–2645. doi:10.1056/NEJMsa022615

McKay, V. R., Morshed, A. B., Brownson, R. C., Proctor, E. K., & Prusaczyk, B. (2018). Letting go: Conceptualizing intervention de-implementation in public health and social service settings. *American Journal of Community Psychology, 62*(1–2), 189–202. doi:10.1002/ajcp.12258

Meier, K. J. (1993). Representative bureaucracy: A theoretical and empirical exposition. *Research in Public Administration, 2*(1), 1–35.

Mohr, L. B. (1982). *Explaining organizational behavior.* San Francisco, CA: Jossey-Bass.

Mosley, J. E., Marwell, N. P., & Ybarra, M. (2019). How the "what works" movement is failing human service organizations, and what social work can do to fix it. *Human Services Organizations: Management, Leadership and Governance.*

National Conference of State Legislatures. (2019). *Family first prevention services act.* Retrieved from http://www.ncsl.org/research/human-services/family-first-prevention-services-act-ffpsa.aspx

National Institutes of Health. (2009). *Dissemination and implementation research in health (R01).* Author. Retrieved from http://grants.nih.gov/grants/guide/pa-files/PAR-10-038.html

Niven, D. J., Mrklas, K. J., Holodinsky, J. K., Straus, S. E., Hemmelgarn, B. R., Jeffs, L. P., & Stelfox, H. T. (2015). Towards understanding the de-adoption of low-value clinical practices: A scoping review. *BMC Medicine, 13.* doi:10.1186/s12916-015-0488-z

Ogden, T., & Fixsen, D. L. (2014). Implementation science. *Zeitschrift Für Psychologie, 222*(1), 4–11. doi:10.1027/2151-2604/a000160

Oliver, C. (1991). Strategic responses to institutional processes. *The Academy of Management Review, 16*(1), 145–179. doi:10.2307/258610

Palinkas, L. A., Holloway, I. W., Rice, E., Fuentes, D., Wu, Q., & Chamberlain, P. (2011). Social networks and implementation of evidence-based practices in public youth-serving systems: A mixed-methods study. *Implementation Science, 6*(1), 113. doi:10.1186/1748-5908-6-113

Palinkas, L. A., & Soydan, H. (2012). *Translation and implementation of evidence-based practice.* New York, NY: Oxford University Press.

Park, S., (Ethan). (2019). Beyond patient-centred care: A conceptual framework of co-production mechanisms with vulnerable groups in health and social service settings. *Public Management Review,* 1–23. doi:10.1080/14719037.2019.1601241

Park, S., (Ethan), Mosley, J. E., & Grogan, C. M. (2016). Do residents of low-income communities trust organizations to speak on their behalf? Differences by organizational type. *Urban Affairs Review, 54*(1), 137–164. doi:10.1177/1078087416669059

Pfeffer, J., & Salancik, G. (1978). *The external control of organizations: A resource dependence perspective.* New York, NY: Harper and Row.

Pinto, R. M., & Witte, S. S. (2019). No easy answers: Avoiding potential pitfalls of de-implementation. *American Journal of Community Psychology, 63*(1–2), 239–242. doi:10.1002/ajcp.12298

Pinto, R. M., Witte, S. S., Filippone, P., Choi, C. J., & Wall, M. (2018a). Interprofessional collaboration and on-the-job training improve access to HIV testing, HIV primary care, and Pre-Exposure Prophylaxis (PrEP). *AIDS Education and Prevention, 30*(6), 474–489. doi:10.1521/aeap.2018.30.6.474

Pinto, R. M., Witte, S. S., Filippone, P. L., Choi, C. J., & Wall, M. (2018b). Policy interventions shaping HIV prevention: Providers' active role in the HIV continuum of care. *Health Education & Behavior, 45*(5), 714–722. doi:10.1177/1090198118760681

Proctor, E. K., Landsverk, J., Aarons, G., Chambers, D., Glisson, C., & Mittman, B. (2009). Implementation research in mental health services: An emerging science with conceptual, methodological, and training challenges. *Administration and Policy in Mental Health, 36,* 1. doi:10.1007/s10488-008-0197-4

Ruef, M. (2000). The emergence of organizational forms: A community ecology approach. *American Journal of Sociology, 106*(3), 658–714. doi:10.1086/318963

US Department of Housing and Urban Development. (2014). *Housing first in permanent supportive housing brief.* Retrieved from https://www.hudexchange.info/resource/3892/housing-first-in-permanent-supportive-housing-brief/

Veniegas, R. C., Kao, U. H., Rosales, R., & Arellanes, M. (2009). HIV prevention technology transfer: Challenges and strategies in the real world. *American Journal of Public Health, 99*(S1), S124–S130. doi:10.2105/AJPH.2007.124263

What Can "Big Data" Methods Offer Human Services Research on Organizations and Communities?

Anna Maria Santiago* and Richard J. Smith*

ABSTRACT

In this commentary, we examine the role that human services professionals might play in the use of Big Data and data science applications that promise to reshape human service organizations and community development activities. We identify what Big Data are and describe the kinds of research that can emanate from Big Data and the use of data science to address contemporary social problems and questions confronting human service organizations and communities. We then discuss existing challenges with the use of Big Data within organizations and communities. We conclude with a discussion of how the larger profession and social work education, specifically, are influenced by the emergence of Big Data and data science techniques.

This commentary on Big Data and data science builds on the themes articulated in the AASWSW Grand Challenge, "Harnessing Technology for Social Good," focusing on implications for research on human service organizations and communities. Recent attention in the popular media has focused on data science applications within child welfare, criminal justice, communications, and political systems; less is known about its use in human service organizations and in community development activities (Kingsley, Coulton, & Pettit, 2014; Tonidandel, King, & Cortina, 2018). This is despite the burgeoning movement toward evidence-based policy and practice that heavily emphasizes the use of data science and Big Data to solve pressing societal problems, a movement which has profound implications on organizational structure and management, budgeting and programmatic decision-making, and how human services will be delivered now and in the future (McNutt, Guo, Goldkind, & An, 2018). As Zetino and Mendoza (2019) note with the call for outcome-based accountability, human services "will be increasingly asked to articulate the value of social services in terms of health, mental health, and 'social determinants' outcomes" (p. 2).

Although the work of the profession is clearly at the forefront of this movement toward information-driven human services, human service professionals are generally absent from the table nor do they inform the decisions that portend to reshape human services programs into the future. Further, the use and potential misuse of data science and Big Data within human services has raised fundamental questions about privacy, the legitimacy of organizational decision-making processes, the lack of representation of marginalized groups and organizations with limited digital access, and the impact on clients and social service delivery systems (Gillingham & Graham, 2017; Goldkind, Thinyane, & Choi, 2018; McNutt et al., 2018). While professional organizations introduced guidance on the use of technology in social work education and practice in 2017, this guidance does not directly address the challenges associated with data science and Big Data in human service organizations and communities

---

*Authors contributed equally to the development of this paper and are thus listed alphabetically.

(National Association of Social Workers, Association of Social Work Boards, Clinical Social Work Association, & Council on Social Work Education, 2017).

In this commentary, we focus on the following questions: What is Big Data? What kind of Big Data research best responds to addressing contemporary social problems? How might Big Data methods tackle previously unknowable questions about human service organizations and communities? What challenges exist for the use of Big Data in human service organizations and communities? What implications does the emergence of Big Data research have on graduate training in social work and other human service professions?

What is Big Data and data science?

"Big Data" refers to datasets that extend "beyond single data repositories and are too large and complex to be processed by traditional database management and methodologies" (Desouza & Smith, 2014, p. 1). The dimensions of Big Data include: volume (i.e., so large the data cannot fit on one server); variety (i.e., structured and unstructured data from different data sources); velocity (i.e., real-time collection and streaming of data from source to user); value (i.e., data provide useful information); volatility (i.e., how long real-time data are valid and should be stored); and veracity (i.e., data integrity protocols are in place)(Bello-Orgaz, Jung, & Camacho, 2016). These data, which require computationally intensive analysis, are stored on networks of distributed servers and are analyzed using specialized software. Moreover, because of their variety and complexity, Big Data paints what Zetino and Mendoza (2019) describe as a "high definition picture of the human experience" (p.1). Yet at the same time, it is important to note that much of these data were not originally collected for research purposes (Connelly, Playford, Gayle, & Dibben, 2016).

Human service managers and professionals are not typically cross-trained as data scientists nor skilled in administering complex data networks. However, they often need to collect, store and analyze vast amounts of administrative data on the clients they serve and are increasingly being asked to make programmatic and funding decisions based on outcomes that may be derived from these data. Therefore, it is important for human service professionals, especially those engaged in management, administration, and community practice to understand the fundamental and radical evolution in data storage, analysis, and usage occurring over the past decade. One fundamental change is in the sheer quantity of data that is constantly updating. The other fundamental change includes new ways of extracting and storing unstructured data that make it easier and more efficient to filter, combine and analyze only the data that is needed. We provide a synthesis of these new Big Data server environments in Table A1, Appendix A.

Data science is the multidisciplinary field developed to analyze Big Data (National Science Foundation, 2019). Traditional social science focuses on hypothesis testing and frequentist inference designed to model the results of randomized clinical trials or random sample survey data. On the other hand, data science focuses on prediction, individualized scenarios, and optimization. Data science is a better fit for human services organizations that rely on administrative data about clients and their communities. Data science, when applied to social science, is typically called computational social science (Russell Sage Foundation, n.d.). Many of the techniques developed for the analysis of Big Data also may be used for large administrative datasets (i.e., 10,000 or more records) and small datasets (i.e., less than 10,000 records). Big Data have the potential to examine complex social phenomenon such as those posed by the 12 Grand Challenges of Social Work. Human services are turning to data science and predictive analytics in order to better target service delivery and improve access to services as well as assess service outcomes (Tonidandel et al., 2018). In particular, Big Data and predictive analytics may help facilitate data sharing and customization of services based on the whole person and their individual needs, proactive intervention in communities through identifying risks to vulnerable populations, and funding decisions based on programmatic outcomes (BCT Partners, 2014; Wareing & Hendrick, 2013). Price (2015) suggests that the use of predictive analytics can ultimately transform human service delivery systems to ones that not only provide transactional services but also make "qualitative changes in people's lives" (para. 3).

How data science could respond to contemporary social problems

Data science methodologies allow for the integration of various types of data that, in turn, enable the study of complex social problems that cannot be addressed using a single data source. These methodologies provide opportunities to examine old research and practice questions in new ways as well as address new questions and emerging areas of practice. Although the use of Big Data for social care and community work has been common in European contexts (especially in Nordic countries), its use has been more limited in the United States. The April 2017 conference entitled, "Grand Challenge to Harness Technology for Social Good" underscores the potential use of Big Data research to address problems related to child welfare, health, housing, and community development. Recent examples of Big Data use in child welfare include the development of a cloud-based child welfare referral system (Curry, van Draanen, & Freisthler, 2017) and the use of predictive analytics for child welfare risk assessment (Cuccaro-Alamin, Foust, Vaithianathan, & Putnam-Hornstein, 2017).

Examples from the NIH's Big Data to Knowledge (BD2K) initiative include the development of mobile apps that have automated intake and behavioral health risk assessments as well as social network analysis of clients in treatment (Walker & Fisman, 2015). Acxiom's Data4Good initiative leverages the use of data to enhance wellness and education in communities (Acxiom, 2014). Wareing and Hendrick (2013) recognize the Home and Healthy for Good Program in Massachusetts as an example of health and human services integration that provides holistic housing and health care for homeless adults (see https://www.mhsa.net/HHG). Vasquez and Barry (2014) describe the use of Testing the Model Approach (TTM) by Chicago LISC partners in improving neighborhood development outcomes in low-income communities. Goldsmith (2014) reports on Buffalo's Operation Clean Sweep Program that uses 311 and 911 calls to identify priority needs and better target services to affected neighborhoods. Johnson (2015) assesses the use of Big Data portals and apps for enhancing the work of community-based organizations in Boston. Other applications of Big Data research include sentiment analysis of social media, geospatial technology, linking data, mobile apps and analyzing streaming data from wearable technology.

Studies by the Center for Urban Poverty and Community Development (see https://case.edu/socialwork/povertycenter/publications) provide an example of best practices in the use of Big Data and data science to enhance community health and well-being. An early leader in the development of integrated datasets to assist community stakeholders to make better decision-making, the Center for Urban Poverty and Community Development (Poverty Center) is part of the National Neighborhood Indicators Partnership – a group of organizations serving 31 cities in the United States (for more information, see https://www.neighborhoodindicators.org). For three decades, the Poverty Center has worked with agencies and organizations forging nontraditional partnerships that led to the creation of NEO CANDO, a neighborhood data warehouse covering 17 counties in Northeast Ohio. NEO CANDO provides free and public access to social and economic data and various mapping and data capturing tools of use to researchers, development professionals, public offices, neighborhood activists, business leaders, and citizens (see http://neocando.case.edu/about-neocando.shtml). Coulton et al. (2010) utilized NEO CANDO data to develop risk models predicting foreclosure risk in metropolitan Cleveland neighborhoods at the height of the Great Recession.

In partnership with Cuyahoga County and other agencies, the Poverty Center created the ChildHood Integrated Longitudinal Data (CHILD) system to facilitate research and evaluation efforts aimed at improving the health and well-being of children in the County (see https://case.edu/socialwork/povertycenter/data-systems/child-data-system). This integrated dataset combines health, education, and child welfare information for children that also was linked to housing and neighborhood data from NEO CANDO. Poverty Center scholars and community partners have examined birth outcomes, child maltreatment, lead exposure and school readiness, homelessness, and juvenile justice involvement using these data systems. Findings to date have been used to make program and policy changes within Cuyahoga County.

How Big Data methods answer questions about human service organizations and communities

Data-driven human services delivery models enable organizations to make real-time decisions to improve services while improving quality of life for families and communities. Big Data applications that link multiple sources of data may facilitate better and more preventative responses to client/community concerns; predict service demands; and enable human service organizations to allocate scarce resources more efficiently (Walker & Fisman, 2015). The availability of Big Data allows organizations to test what works, assess programmatic outcomes or impacts of the work that they do, and weigh the benefits vs. the costs of programs and services. Fruchterman (2016, p. 1) suggests that data make "the work of social change agents more effective" and "build support for best practices." Table 1 summarizes these questions and methods. A data science approach typically prefers data in a graphical form as opposed to tables or text (i.e., a *data visualization*). Several data visualizations often are presented together in near real-time on an online dashboard accessible on any mobile device. See Appendix Table A3 for more information.

Big Data methods are used to classify information, an aspect of artificial intelligence that is key to human services applications. For example, *machine learning*, uses a training dataset (e.g., a subset) to find the best model to fit the data that is then used on a larger dataset. Spam email filters and speech recognition use machine learning. In *supervised learning*, analysts inspect the output and update model parameters. However, some machine learning algorithms are *unsupervised* and cross-validated automatically. In computational social science, machine learning (e.g., *support vector machines*) can be used to predict multiple categories and in turn be used to match treatment and comparison groups for a quasi-experimental design (e.g., using the GenMatch package in R). Machine learning also may be used to analyze and classify text and images (e.g., deep learning, neural networks). For example, Smith (2015) used machine learning to match comparison neighborhoods to test the impact of the Empowerment Zone program. In this Federal program from the 1990s, HUD designated some high poverty neighborhoods to receive a combination of tax incentives and grants. Machine learning made it possible to find the best set of comparison neighborhoods from a larger

Table 1. Computational social science questions and methods for macro social work.

Subfield	Questions	Computational social science methods
Community Indicators	How do we know if the look and feel of a neighborhood is changing over time? (Glaeser, Kominers, Luca, & Naik, 2018; Kingsley et al., 2014)	Imagery analysis, classification, machine-learning
Neighborhood Change	How do we know which neighborhoods are at risk of decline or gentrification? (Greene & Pettit, 2016)	Predictive analytics, classification, machine-learning
Community Health	How can we measure community well-being in real time? (Bresnick, 2017; Gamache, Kharrazi, & Weiner, 2018)	Web scraping, social media scraping, machine learning, classification
Housing and Community Development	How do low-income families classify over time in terms of residential contextual mobility? (Lee, Smith, & Galster, 2017)	Sequence analysis
Management and Administration	How can we support risk assessment? (Cuccaro-Alamin et al., 2017; Zabinski et al., 2018)	Predictive analytics, support vector machines, Bayesian network modeling
Policy Practice	How do we understand the social construction of policy, or the role of advocacy coalitions in the passage of policy? (Giest, 2017)	Web scraping, automated text analysis with machine learning

pool. However, this was a supervised approach, which meant that each match had to be assessed for balance before proceeding to calculating the impact of the tax incentives on jobs.

On the other hand, in research on complex, dynamic systems, researchers may now use Bayesian Network Modeling (e.g., bnlearn) as an unsupervised learning approach to causal inference. Recently, an interdisciplinary team used unsupervised Bayesian Network Models to predict Ebola virus outbreaks at wastewater treatment plants (Zabinski, Pieper, & Gibson, 2018). As input variables, the model takes data on Ebola patients from hospitals, disinfectant levels, water temperature, and more to predict risk to workers who treat water. The advantage of an unsupervised approach is that real-time changes can be processed automatically. However, as with any automatic process, the model and results need to be interpreted with caution.

Social media has expanded the field of social network analysis and graph analytics. With a focus on predictive analytics, data analysis using Big Data utilizes *data mining* in order to find patterns within data. The use of *association rules*, an example of a supervised algorithm (e.g., aRules in R), enables analysts to estimate the probability of a particular service use given prior service utilization. This algorithm is the one used by Amazon.com to recommend other products for people to buy given past purchases. For example, if you buy one book on social work research (e.g., Auerbach & Zeitlin, 2015), Amazon.com will suggest other social work books based on the conditional probabilities of every other shopper. What online retailers have in common with human service organizations is that they are making decisions based on administrative or other self-selected samples. That is why Big Data analysts use Bayesian inference to calculate conditional probabilities, which achieves the goal of predicting individual behavior given the available data. These types of prediction may or may not involve theory or hypothesis testing because there is no need to generalize outside of the customer base. In human services, this could be used to suggest services to clients, but we would not recommend making these suggestions mandatory.

Additionally, analysis of the Twitter firehose has been used to create a method called *sentiment analysis*; recent social work research has used this approach to assess neighborhood-level psychological distress (Booth, Lin, & Wei, 2018). In this example, Booth, et al. analyzed social media tweets qualitatively for themes related to psychometric states using a published lexicon. They created a neighborhood level variable based on the tweets originating in each neighborhood and found that high poverty neighborhoods are associated with tweets expressing sentiments of psychological distress. This Big Data analysis can be used to target prevention work.

Challenges for use of Big Data in human service organizations and communities

As Desouza and Smith (2014) note, the gap between the potential of Big Data and actual use by human service organizations to address social problems is considerable. Currently, most data held in individual human service organizations limit data sharing across organizations – even those providing the same or similar services. At the outset, most human service organizations have limited staffing and resources, and inadequate infrastructure to store and protect data. Additionally, administrative data collected in agency settings are often inaccessible – captured on paper or in other formats that render data analyses difficult at best. Except in some of the larger human service organizations, there is a lack of dedicated staff trained in data entry and verification. As a result, existing staff members with little or no data entry training are asked to assume these tasks in addition to providing services, which often results in missing and/or incomplete data in organizational databases.

These concerns are magnified by the values and choices made by individuals who design and analyze the datasets; Big Data decision-making and algorithm construction are not neutral activities. *How well can predictive analytics handle extremely rare events in an environment with missing data, disparities, and bias?* The lack of in-house data analysts or the ability to hire outside consultants hinders an organization's ability to utilize administrative data for programmatic and funding decisions. Moreover, the lack of policies and cooperative agreements establishing and regulating the use of Big Data limits the ability of human service organizations to offer more comprehensive, person-centered services since the full array of client concerns and access to existing service delivery systems remains unknown.

Additionally, the risk of predictive analytics applied to human services settings, like child welfare and health care, raise serious ethical issues about privacy and data veracity (Cuccaro-Alamin et al., 2017; Tonidandel et al., 2018; Yampolskaya, 2017). In a recent article, Heeks and Renken (2018) underscore multiple data practices that undermine the rights of clients in human services organizations. These include surveillance, the loss of privacy and algorithmic profiling. For example, a health NGO obtained access to detailed mobile phone data without consent of the individual client. In this data mining example, the principles of access, privacy and inclusion are violated. Heeks and Renken (2018) argue that professionals working in organizations and communities need to incorporate practices that support the fair use and handling of data as well as the rights of data access, ownership and representation or inclusion.

In response to some of the aforementioned concerns, social workers and other human service professionals have new guidance on the use of technology in education, research, and practice (Berzin, Singer, & Chan, 2015; Heeks & Renken, 2018; National Association of Social Workers et al., 2017). These standards apply social work values of privacy, confidentiality, autonomy and access. However, much of the discussion is about setting boundaries (e.g., social media) or protecting private data about clients (e.g., encrypting devices). There is standard cautioning for social workers to understand "open data," how the use of data could affect clients and some language about online research. However, one of the innovations in Big Data research is to use metadata as a predictor. Even if social workers maintain separate social media identities for clients and clients have separate social media identities for interacting with their social workers, these metadata from both be aggregated and sold to marketing firms. Further, many social media sites ask users to agree to turn over all their data to the U.S. government upon request. In both scenarios, clients could be reidentified.

One of the limitations of Big Data is its representativeness. What kind of selection bias exists in administrative data? Or social media data? Coupled with concerns about representativeness are concerns about replicability. To what extent are Big Data findings reproducible if the data are constantly changing? Finally, given differential access to both data and information technology, there are concerns about the extent to which organizations and communities may experience "digital redlining," or the creation of hierarchies of access whereby organizations and communities with the fewest resources will be excluded from the benefits that may accrue from less restricted access to Big Data and its associated technologies.

What is the role of human service scholars and professionals in addressing ethical considerations in the use of Big Data and data science?

Social work's commitment to social justice has a logical extension in advocacy for data justice for individual clients with the organizations that serve them. In other words, human service professionals can play a strong role in shaping individual and societal norms regarding the use of data including the capacity to make informed choices regarding opting in or out of participation. Our work across organizations and communities can help facilitate careful examination of the potential uses and abuses of administrative data. We need to be at the table in order to consider both the ethical and social implications of technologies as they are developed. We also need to advocate for the development of policies regulating the responsible use of data science techniques for research and innovation. Once such policy might be modeled after the European Union's General Data Protection Regulation that was passed in May 2018. Specifically, Article 22(1) stipulates the right of people not to be subject to a decision based solely on automated processing. With the advent of practices requiring data-driven human services decision-making, professionals in social work and human services need to be mindful of making programmatic and funding decisions that consider data beyond those that are mined using data science techniques.

Implications for graduate training in social work and human services professions

Currently, social work and human services graduate students (and faculty) need to be prepared to handle Big Data, especially in terms of the information technologies required to use them. Big Data centers and institutes need to have social work faculty or students on staff. As experienced graduate faculty, the authors are well aware of variations in experience and comfort levels with Big Data and tools to analyze it. One might ask, why teach Big Data if it is a struggle to teach small data? One reason might be the mismatch between the questions frequentist statistics can answer and the data practitioners have in the field. As noted earlier, data visualization offers a more initiative way of understanding client and organizational performance.

Several social work programs have started training students in data science. One of the leading centers training social welfare doctoral students in Big Data applications is the Guizhou UC-Berkeley Big Data Innovation Research Center (GBIC) (Berkeley Social Welfare, n.d.). The Maryland Longitudinal Data Systems Center (n.d.) at the School of Social Work provides dashboards and research services for state education and workforce agencies (University of Maryland, n.d.). For the past several years, the Silberman School of Social Work at Hunter College has been hosting an annual summer institute in computational social science. This institute brings together doctoral students from all over the country to Harlem to learn programming in R, to do data visualization, web scraping, text analysis, and machine learning. Additionally, the University of Pennsylvania School of Policy and Practice recently developed a data analytics certificate for policy students. Nonetheless, these training opportunities have yet to become mainstream in the profession. Other social work programs, such as the School of Social Work at the University of Toronto, have partnered with schools of information or business to provide training in data science. Finally, a number of university programs and centers (e.g., the Center for Artificial Intelligence in Society co-founded by Eric Rice, a faculty member at the USC Suzanne Dworak-Peck School of Social Work; the University of Michigan Child and Adolescent Data Lab; or Partners for Our Children at the University of Washington) could be identified with the larger Data4Good movement (see Howson, 2018). By sponsoring initiatives aimed at making data science applications accessible to human service organizations in underserved communities, these entities help to level the playing field.

Students need interdisciplinary training that is intentional and not just a few cognate courses. In other words, training needs to include interprofessional opportunities to participate in research collaborations with health professionals, other social scientists, engineers, and natural scientists. Finally, graduate programs in social work and the human services should encourage the submission of NSF dissertation improvement grants for basic science research using Big Data applications. Professionals in social work and the human services are well positioned to contribute to the conversation about broader public impacts of Big Data research as well as to lead community engagement. NSF is the key funder of interdisciplinary Big Data research and data science and if social work wants to be part of this conversation, that is one place to go. The Russell Sage Foundation, the foundation that provided the startup capital for formal social work education, also funds Big Data research as part of its Computational Social Science program. The foundation focuses on funding research that links administrative data in new ways or uses Big Data methods to analyze large volumes of qualitative information.

Coulton, Goerge, Putnam-Hornstein, and de Haan (2015) contend that social work programs need to teach Bayesian inference in addition to frequentist statistics to enhance quantitative analysis. Likewise, research methodologies that facilitate the analysis of unstructured data will support both qualitative and quantitative research. Doctoral programs in social work and human services need to train students how to work with these methods if they are to be competitive for future funding. Table 2 presents a side-by-side comparison of one possible Big Data curriculum relative to a typical doctoral curriculum. One could imagine this in lieu of a traditional curriculum or perhaps in addition to a traditional doctoral curriculum. At the very least, social work researchers need to know how to program in R and Python, as much as they program using

Table 2. Potential data science social work doctoral curriculum.

	Typical social work methods curriculum	Social work + Big Data
Fall 1	• Descriptive and Bivariate Statistics • Research Design, Ethics, and Philosophy	• Computer environments (Programming in R and Python using GitHub, NoSQL, Apache, Hadoop) • Research design and ethics • Statistics for data science (Distinguishing, Bayesian, Frequentist, Liklihoodist)
Winter 1	• Multivariate Statistics (OLS, GLM) • Research Methods, Survey Design, Instrumentation • Qualitative Methods	• Data mining (text analysis, web-scraping, imagery analysis, sentiment analysis) • Causal inference + Machine learning (Support vector machines, association rules, genetic algorithms) • Research project management
Fall 2	• Advanced Statistics (Longitudinal/SEM/Multilevel Methods) • Mixed Methods/Program Evaluation/Community Based Participatory Action Research	• Advanced Statistics (Longitudinal/SEM/Multilevel Methods) • Advanced Machine Learning (Bayesian Network modeling, neural networks, deep learning)
Winter 2	• Methods Electives (e.g., survival analysis, GIS)	• Data visualization • Methods Electives

SAS, Stata, or SPSS. Some of the qualitative data software, such as QDA Miner, have integrated data mining, web scraping and automated text analysis using machine learning into their existing menus. There are machine learning packages written for Stata as well. Social work faculty and students need to know how to work in a secure server environment. Ethics associated with data integrity and privacy need to be infused throughout the curriculum.

Many of these suggestions are unlikely to be implemented in social work education, but we can start small by understanding the ethical challenges of Big Data and learn the most relevant techniques in order to harness this technology for social good.

Conclusions

Big Data and data science are revolutionizing the ways human service organizations and management (HSO&M) researchers conduct research. Deans and Associate Deans for Research may be unprepared for the speed at which data science is changing research agendas. At bare minimum, HSO&M researchers should employ more robust ways of conducting intervention studies that rely on quasi-experimental design. However, data science also gives HSO&M researchers a better window into social problems. HSO&M researchers should use these improved algorithms to classify people, organizations, and places based on structured or unstructured data. This could potentially disrupt classifications derived from an institutional process, like the Diagnostic and Statistical Manual. One question that researchers could answer would be to see if unstructured methods to analyze text of intake interviews and case notes could improve diagnosis, treatment planning, and results. HSO&M researchers could also ask how human service organizations cluster based on their mission or program characteristics described in tax reporting. For example, do these classifications match the National Taxonomy of Exempt Entities (NTEE) Codes (e.g., Children & Youth Services, Senior Centers, Ethnic & Immigrant Centers)?

In terms of organizational research problems, HSO&M researchers could work with near real-time performance data aligned with logic model outcomes. We have the technology to build a real-time dashboard for each client, each human services worker, and each human services manager. Research could determine how realistic it is for human service workers and managers to enter data and check a dashboard to make decisions. Finally, communities are changing rapidly. HSO&M

researchers can use research to predict real estate prices and use these predictions to prevent segregation, housing discrimination, gentrification, displacement, or eviction. Ultimately, however, these phenomena are shaped by deliberate policy decisions. Is it realistic to think that having access to more data would change vested interests?

Data science has the potential to predict an event before it happens. HSO&M researchers will need to decide if this can be done ethically and how to protect rights. From a data science perspective, predicting a suicide, for example, is just a matter of having enough. One could imagine an intervention trial of a mobile app that uses data from a client's location, activity level, purchases, and social media posts to monitor progress toward a treatment plan. We can predict smog to issue a "spare the air day alert." Can we use Big Data to issue a "spare a life" alert for instances when child abuse, suicide, or intimate partner violence peak? This is no easy task, as further research is needed on the ethical use of data, especially when data are from private sources.

To what extent will researchers and practitioners in human services organizations and social work seize the opportunities afforded by access to these data and methodologies to enhance the work we do? We hope that these professions will accept the benefits while acknowledging the challenges of these approaches in order to improve the quality of life of individuals, families, and communities.

Disclosure statement

No potential conflict of interest was reported by the authors.

References

Acxiom. (2014 September 24). Acxiom launches program to leverage its data power for community wellness. Retrieved from: https://www.businesswire.com/news/home/20140923005114/en/Acxiom-Launches-Program-Leverage-Data-Power-Community

Auerbach, C., & Zeitlin, W. (2015). Making your case: Using R for program evaluation. Oxford, England, UK: Oxford University Press.

BCT Partners. (2014 March 28). Three ways big data can reshape social programs. Retrieved from https://www.bctpartners.com/single-post/2018/03/28/Three-Ways-Big-Data-Can-Reshape-Social-Programs

Bello-Orgaz, G., Jung, J. J., & Camacho, D. (2016). Social big data: Recent achievements and new challenges. Information Fusion, 28, 45–59. doi:10.1016/j.inffus.2015.08.005

Berkeley Social Welfare. (n.d.). Guizhou Berkeley big data innovation research center. Retrieved from https://socialwelfare.berkeley.edu/gbic

Berzin, S. C., Singer, J., & Chan, C. (2015). Practice innovation through technology in the digital age: A grand challenge for social work. Cleveland, Ohio: American Academy of Social Work and Social Welfare.

Booth, J. M., Lin, Y.-R., & Wei, K. (2018). Neighborhood disadvantage, residents' distress, and online social communication: Harnessing Twitter data to examine neighborhood effects. Journal of Community Psychology, 46(7), 829–843. doi:10.1002/jcop.22094

Bresnick, J. (2017, March 29). Big data analytics link economic wellness to population health. Retrieved from https://healthitanalytics.com/news/big-data-analytics-link-economic-wellness-to-population-health

Connelly, R., Playford, C. J., Gayle, V., & Dibben, C. (2016). The role of administrative data in the big data revolution in social science research. Social Science Research, 59, 1–12. doi:10.1016/j.ssresearch.2016.04.015

Coulton, C., Hexter, K. W., Hirsh, A., O'Shaughnessy, A., Richter, F. G. C., & Schramm, M. (2010). Facing the foreclosure crisis in Greater Cleveland: What happened and how communities are responding. Federal Reserve Bank of Cleveland, Urban Publications, Paper 374, 01. 01.2010.

Coulton, C. J., Goerge, R., Putnam-Hornstein, E., & de Haan, B. (2015). Harnessing big data for social good: A grand challenge for social work (Vol. 11, pp. 21). Cleveland, Ohio: American Academy of Social Work and Social Welfare. Retrieved from https://aaswsw.org/wp-content/uploads/2015/07/Big-Data-GC-edited-and-formatted-for-committee-review-7-17-20151.pdf

Cuccaro-Alamin, S., Foust, R., Vaithianathan, R., & Putnam-Hornstein, E. (2017). Risk assessment and decision making in child protective services: Predictive risk modeling in context. Children and Youth Services Review, 79, 291–298. doi:10.1016/j.childyouth.2017.06.027

Curry, S. R., van Draanen, J., & Freisthler, B. (2017). Perceptions and use of a web-based referral system in child welfare: Differences by caseworker tenure. Journal of Technology in Human Services, 35(2), 152–168. doi:10.1080/15228835.2017.1330725

Desouza, K. C., & Smith, K. L. (2014, Summer). Big data for social innovation. *Stanford Social Innovation Review*, *2014*, 39–43.

Fruchterman, J. (2016, Summer). Using data for action and for impact. *Stanford Social Innovation Review, 2016*, 30–35.

Gamache, R., Kharrazi, H., & Weiner, J. (2018). Public and population health informatics: The bridging of big data to benefit communities. *Yearbook of Medical Informatics, 27*(01), 199–206. doi:10.1055/s-0038-1667081

Giest, S. (2017). Big data for policymaking: Fad or fasttrack? *Policy Sciences, 50*(3), 367–382. doi:10.1007/s11077-017-9293-1

Gillingham, P., & Graham, T. (2017). Big data in social welfare: The development of a critical perspective on social work's latest "electronic turn". *Australian Social Work, 70*(2), 135–147. doi:10.1080/0312407X.2015.1134606

Glaeser, E. L., Kominers, S. D., Luca, M., & Naik, N. (2018). Big data and big cities: The promises and limitations of improved measures of urban life. *Economic Inquiry, 56*(1), 114–137. doi:10.1111/ecin.12364

Goldkind, L., Thinyane, M., & Choi, M. (2018). Small data, big justice: The intersection of data science, social good and social services. *Journal of Technology in Human Services, 36*, 175–178. doi:10.1080/15228835.2018.1539369

Goldsmith, S. (2014, February 11). Big data gives a boost to health and human services. Retrieved from https://datasmart.ash.harvard.edu/news/article/big-data-gives-a-boost-to-health-and-human-services.html

Greene, S., & Pettit, K. L. S. (2016). *What if cities used data to drive inclusive neighborhood change?* Retrieved from Urban Institute website: http://www.urban.org/sites/default/files/publication/81306/2000807-What-if-Cities-Used-Data-to-Drive-Inclusive-Neighborhood-Change.pdf

Heeks, R., & Renken, J. (2018). Data justice for development: What would it mean? *Information Development, 34*, 90–102. doi:10.1177/0266666916678282

Howson, C. (2018 June 23). Data for good: Movement or moment? *Information Management*. Retrieved from https://www.information-management.com/opinion/data-for-good-movement-or-moment

Johnson, M. P. (2015). Data, analytics and community-based organizations: Transforming data to decisions for community development. *ISJLP, 11*, 49.

Kingsley, G. T., Coulton, C. J., & Pettit, K. L. S. (2014). *Strengthening communities with neighborhood data*. Washington D.C.: Urban Institute Press.

Lee, K. O., Smith, R., & Galster, G. (2017). Subsidized housing and residential trajectories: An application of matched sequence analysis. *Housing Policy Debate, 27*(6), 843–874. doi:10.1080/10511482.2017.1316757

Maryland Longitudinal Data System Center. (n.d.). MLDSC Home. Retrieved from https://mldscenter.maryland.gov/welcome-index.html

McNutt, J., Guo, C., Goldkind, L., & An, S. (2018). *Technology in nonprofit organizations and voluntary action*. Leiden, NL: Brill.

National Association of Social Workers, Association of Social Work Boards, Clinical Social Work Association, & Council on Social Work Education. (2017). *Standards for technology in social work practice*. Retrieved from https://www.socialworkers.org/includes/newIncludes/homepage/PRA-BRO-33617.TechStandards_FINAL_POSTING.pdf

National Science Foundation. (2019, February 11). Harnessing the data revolution (HDR): Transdisciplinary research in principles of data science phase I. Retrieved from https://www.nsf.gov/pubs/2019/nsf19550/nsf19550.htm

Price, M. (2015 October 30). From transactional to transformative: Rethinking human services delivery. Retrieved from https://blogs.deloitte.com/centerforhealthsolutions/from-transactional-to-transformative-rethinking-human-services-delivery/

Russell Sage Foundation. (n.d.). Computational social science. Retrieved from http://www.russellsage.org/special-initiatives/computational-social-science

Smith, R. (2015). Empowerment for whom? The impact of community renewal tax incentives on jobs and businesses. *Urban Studies, 52*(4), 702–720. doi:10.1177/0042098014528398

Tonidandel, S., King, E. B., & Cortina, J. M. (2018). Big data methods: Leveraging modern data analytic techniques to build organizational science. *Organizational Research Methods, 21*(3), 525–547. doi:10.1177/1094428116677299

Vasquez, S., & Barry, P. (2014). *Everything old is new again: Building nonprofit capacity in the age of big data*. Retrieved from http://www.whatcountsforamerica.org/portfolio/427/

Walker, B., & Fisman, T. (2015). *Rethinking human services delivery: Using data-driven insights for transformational outcomes*. Deloitte Consulting. Retrieved from https://www2.deloitte.com/insights/us/en/industry/public-sector/human-services-delivery-data-driven-insights.html

Wareing, T., & Hendrick, H. H. (2013, April 1). 5 trends driving the future of human services. Retrieved from https://www.govtech.com/health/5-Trends-Driving-the-Future-of-Human-Services.html

Yampolskaya, S. (2017). Administrative data and behavioral science research. *Families in Society, 98*, 121–125. doi:10.1606/1044-3894.2017.98.17

Zabinski, J. W., Pieper, K. J., & Gibson, J. M. (2018). A Bayesian belief network model assessing the risk to wastewater workers of contracting ebola virus disease during an outbreak. *Risk Analysis, 38*(2), 376–391. doi:10.1111/risa.2018.38.issue-2

Zetino, J., & Mendoza, N. (2019). Big data and its utility in social work: Learning from the Big Data revolution in business and healthcare. *Social Work in Public Health, 34*(5), 409–417. doi:10.1080/19371918.2019.1614508

Appendix A. Big Data Environments

Table A1 provides a synthesis of these new Big Data server environments. These are software that sit in the cloud or on local servers to facilitate storage, cleaning, and access. A new set of programming languages (e.g., R, Python, Pig Latin among others) have evolved to organize, clean and analyze Big Data (See Table A2). Big Data tools include data wrangling libraries (e.g., data extracting, cleaning and reshaping) and allow for the extraction and analysis of unstructured text, images, and numbers from various Internet sources. They also include software for data visualization (See Table A3).

Table A1. Big Data server environments and implications for social work.

Name	Type	Purpose	Training potential for social work
Apache Hadoop (https://hadoop.apache.org/)	Software Library Framework for Big Data	Allows Big Data to be distributed, stored and analyzed across different servers.	Minimal: Requires extensive cross training or partnering.
MapReduce (https://hadoop.apache.org/)	Programming model	Filter, sort, and process Big Data across multiple servers.	Minimal.
Apache Spark (https://spark.apache.org/)	Cluster computing framework	Allows data to be analyzed in the cloud.	Minimal.
NoSQL(http://nosql-database.org/)	Database	Data are stored as columns, documents, graphs, key-values or in other ways to accommodate unstructured data in the cloud.	NoSQL and other methods of storing and analyzing unstructured data can be readily introduced in training programs.

Table A2. Data science programming languages and software.

Name	Type	Purpose	Training potential for social work
R (https://cran.r-project.org/)	Statistical Programming Language	Data analysis	R is essential for social work research. Auerbach and Zeitlin (2015) have specific R textbooks for macro social workers.
RStudio (https://www.rstudio.com/)	Integrated Development Environment	Desktop software for writing, executing and visualizing data using the R programming language.	The preferred environment for writing and running R programs.
Python (https://www.python.org/)	Programming language	Data analysis with particular strengths in matrix algebra, text, and imagery analysis.	Python is an essential tool for social work researchers who use geographic data.
iPython Notebooks (https://ipython.org/notebook.html)	Interactive computational environment	Software that can reside on a desktop or cloud to write software, preview results, and run programs.	This is the preferred environment for writing and running Python programs.
Apache Pig + Pig Latin (https://pig.apache.org/)	Platform that runs on Hadoop with programming language called Pig Latin	Send commands on Hadoop to MapReduce and Spark.	Requires extensive cross training or partnering.
GitHub (https://github.com/)	Software for programming collaboration with version tracking.	Allows team members to collaborate on different parts of code writing in the cloud with a desktop client. They can fork and then merge different parts of a project. Integrates with RStudio.	For big and small data projects, GitHub is the preferred way to do reproducible and collaborative research.

Table A3. Data visualization.

Name	Type	Purpose	Training potential for social work
D3: Data Driven Documents (https://d3js.org/)	JavaScript library	Visualize Big Data online.	Good online library for inspiration but would require ability to program in Java.
Gephi (https://gephi.org/)	Open Source Desktop Software	Visualize social network data.	This is suitable for a brief overview of social networks for a social work class to teach how individuals and organizations are connected.
ggplot2 (https://ggplot2.tidyverse.org/)	R package	One of R's leading data visualization packages based on the Grammar of Graphics. Can visualize trends and different categorical variables simultaneously.	If you teach R, teaching ggplot2 and other tidyverse packages would be essential for social work research.
Microsoft Excel (https://products.office.com/en-us/excel)	Proprietary desktop office application	Make basic plots with small or medium sized database or stream Big Data from cloud.	Every graduate professional needs to know how to use a spreadsheet application.
Raw (https://rawgraphs.io/)	Online data visualization website	Visualize data online – big or small.	Simple interface ready for a social work classroom. Can cut and paste data or stream it using a URL. Not for restricted data unless the software is copied to a secure computer.
Tableau (https://public.tableau.com/s/)	Proprietary software with no cost version	Visualize data from a spreadsheet or from cloud. Integrates with Excel, R.	A reasonable choice for a BSW/MSW macro social work curriculum, but it may take extensive reshaping of spreadsheets. Must purchase a license if using restricted data.

Note: Line graphs make it easy to show both human service workers and managers if client trends are improving. Dot charts and bar graphs can be used by analysts if different categories have different sizes. Maps of places and relationships are also useful visualizations.

Crafting the Future of Macro Practice

John Tropman and Bowen McBeath

ABSTRACT

This Discussion of the Special Issue addresses four interlocking questions of importance for social work macro practice: (1) What is the trajectory of macro practice in schools of social work?; (2) What should be included in a 21st century macro practice curriculum?; (3) How can schools of social work promote research on organizations, managers, and leaders; and (4) What under-explored research topics in organizational and management practice exist? The Discussion links major themes among the 10 commentaries comprising the Special Issue in order to provide some perspective on longstanding concerns to social work scholars. In essence, we transition from a discussion of the commentaries, to situating the concerns of the commentaries in the social work academy. Our central argument is that calls for a strengthening of social work macro practice education and research should be directed at deans and directors. Yet deans of schools of social work are middle managers within complex academic institutional hierarchies. They must regularly compete and collaborate with other deans for resources, interest, and status. Thus, it is incumbent upon macro practice educators and researchers to clearly demonstrate what macro practice education and research do for schools of social work vis-à-vis other professional schools and universities. If macro practice professors cannot argue convincingly and succinctly for their investments in more public fora, then deans and directors may not either. Our argument holds for academic innovators in competitive knowledge industries as much as it does for social entrepreneurs and organizational leaders in competitive human service industries.

For several years, social work researchers invested in organizational and management issues have met at the Society for Social Work Research (SSWR) Annual Conference to discuss the state of macro practice. These discussions have focused upon the following questions, among others:

(1) *Macro practice trajectory.* What is the trajectory of macro practice in schools of social work, and particularly in relation to organizations and management?
(2) *Content of macro practice curriculum.* What do we want a macro practice curriculum to include? What is missing from the existing curriculum, and what new or ignored knowledge would be beneficial?
(3) *A research desert?* Why is there less investment in research on organizational, management, and leadership practice in schools of social work?
(4) *Emerging problems and prospects.* What unexplored and under-explored problem areas and opportunities exist in management and leadership research?

In anticipation of a workgroup meeting at the January 2019 SSWR Annual Conference, distinguished members of SSWR were invited to write commentaries on the future of human service organizational and management (HSO&M) research. The 10 commentaries presented in this special issue are a result of that invitation. Each commentary related directly to the four questions noted above.

This discussion links major themes among the commentaries, highlighted in the introduction to the special issue, with some perspective on longstanding concerns to scholars within schools of social work. In essence, the goal is to transition from a discussion of the commentaries, to situating the concerns of the commentaries in the social work academy.

Our central claim is that calls for a strengthening of social work macro practice education and research should be directed at deans and directors. Yet deans of schools of social work are middle managers within complex academic institutional hierarchies. They must regularly compete and collaborate with other deans for resources, interest, and status. Thus, it is incumbent upon macro practice educators and researchers to clearly demonstrate what macro practice education and research do for schools of social work vis-à-vis other professional schools and universities. If faculty members cannot provide such information in middle management terms – e.g., academic return on investment, data integration and data dashboards – then future requests for macro practice education and research may be viewed less sympathetically.

Therefore, we would argue that macro practice professors should view their educational and research initiatives from a perspective of venture capitalism, by combining brief story-based explanations for the centrality of their contributions allied to the use of qualitative and quantitative data to demonstrate their promise (if not their effectiveness). Consider, for example, that SSWR has increasingly experimented with "brief and brilliant" sessions at the Annual Conference, which reflect the use of TED Talks. If macro practice professors cannot argue convincingly and succinctly for their investments in more public fora, then deans and directors may not either. Our argument holds for academic innovators in competitive knowledge industries as much as it does for social entrepreneurs and HSO&M leaders in competitive human service industries. We elaborate upon the basic logic of our argument in the following brief sections, which correspond with the four questions listed above.

What is the trajectory of macro practice in schools of social work?

It has been argued that social work macro practice is not as strong as it could be. This argument is not a new one, and has spanned generations going back before the rise of the behavioral revolution in the social sciences. For example, recent macro practice-focused conversations are predated by an historic question of whether social work is a profession (Flexner, 1915; Specht & Courtney, 1995). More recently, statistics from the Council on Social Work Education (CSWE) indicated that there are 862 programs across all levels of study, containing 127,079 students (CSWE, 2016). Just under half of programs (47%) were BSW programs, which are almost exclusively generalist and likely contain extremely modest macro content.

Table 1. MSW student enrollment by practice specialization/concentration.

Student Specializations in MSW Study	Number of Students	Percentage
Clinical/Direct Practice	20,157	62.66
Advanced Generalist	7,183	22.33
Other	2,598	8.08
Macro Practice		
Community Organizing, Planning, and Development	1,112	3.46
Administration	880	2.49
Policy Practice	197	0.61
Nonprofit/Public Management	100	0.31
Evaluation	20	0.06
Total	32,167	100

Student statistics reflect 2015 data (CSWE, 2016).

At the MSW level and as can be seen in Table 1, available data from MSW programs suggested that small proportions of students were majoring in macro areas (with over two-thirds in clinical/direct practice and advanced generalists practice concentrations) (CSWE, 2016). These data certainly show the low volume of macro practice education, a point that commentators of the special issue stressed repeatedly.

With respect to Ph.D. and DSW programs, the numbers are small – a point to be discussed later in regards to the hope for future research on HSO&M. But we can assume that the macro practice vs. non-macro practice proportions at the doctoral level are reasonably close to the MSW breakdown. Thus, the overall numbers and percentages of macro practice students seem to be exceptionally limited, which is bad news for the field.

As implied in the commentaries (notably Austin and Hoefer), schools of social work seem to be failing to do their macro practice duty, especially in BSW (generalist) programs but also in most MSW programs. Analysis of such lacunae must start with the deans and directors, and not only those who are currently in their posts but also their predecessors. In terms of its eschewal of macro practice leadership, it can be argued that CSWE has sidestepped or avoided leadership in terms of its commitment to "field of practice diversity, equity, and inclusion". Finally, the community of professional HSO&M executives (with a key exception to be mentioned later) has failed to challenge the social work education and training community to take a more "macroscopic" view and macro practice-oriented posture.

In their outward-facing role, social work leaders need to recognize and embrace the importance of management and leadership in our sector – not as a peripheral afterthought but as a central part of the sector. We need to get outside of our workplaces, engage with civic associations and councils of health and human service organizations, and join with other community groups. To develop leader and managers, we need to initiate and staff a "Better Community Benefit Organization Bureau" to fill the gap left by the demise of the Councils of Social Agencies (similar to how the Better Business Bureau represents local businesses).

As schools of social work have missed opportunities to expand macro practice education, research, and service, other sources of HSO&M education and training have emerged – particularly, nonprofit management centers. These centers, usually on the smaller scale and often embedded within schools of public policy, management, and business, provide education and training for students and community leaders interested in the nonprofit sector. To some extent, schools of social work have ceded nonprofit leadership education and training at the degree/professional level to other academic units.

Loose coordination is provided by the Nonprofit Academic Centers Council (NACC), whose mission statement includes:

"At universities across the nation, dedicated students and nonprofit professionals are seeking the knowledge they need to make an impact on the nonprofit sector and the world. Responding to this demand, more than 255 colleges and universities provide at least one class in nonprofit management, including 157 schools that offer at least one course within a graduate department. On these campuses and others, centers for the study of philanthropy and nonprofit organizations are a focal point for diverse disciplines to combine thoughtful scholarship with practical applications" (Nonprofit Academic Centers Council, 2019).

Of the 50 member programs constituting the NACC, only one is housed within a school of social work (The Mandel School at Case Western Reserve University).

This imbalance reveals another gap: post-MSW (and other advanced degreed) leadership and management education. With the exception of a few social work executive leadership programs (including at the University of Michigan, the University of California-Berkeley, and Hunter College-CUNY), executive education programs at schools of social work are largely absent. In contrast, there is no significant business school that does not have an executive education division. However, it is important to note that few business executives dedicate sufficient time and funds for education. Nor do HSO&M leaders or schools of social work invest sufficiently. They do not like to pay for staff development, so the professional cadre is undereducated.

As an exception to the rule, the University of Michigan Executive Leadership Program (ELP) has been in existence for 19 years. The ELP is a unique partnership among the School of Social Work, the Ross School of Business, and the Alliance for Strong Families and Communities (which is a national alliance of state and local associations of leading child and family serving agencies). Aside from some agency arrangements at the University of Notre Dame Business School under the leadership of its former director Tom Harvey (previously the CEO of Catholic Charities USA), the ELP is the only program where a school of social work has partnered with a national association to provide executive education for its member agencies.

A future opportunity thus may exist for academic-practice partnerships focused upon executive education. Specifically, the Network for Social Work Management (with its roughly 15,000 members worldwide) has been in existence for about 30 years, and has developed a management/leadership certificate program in which MSW students can be certified if their macro practice concentrations incorporate sufficient curricular attention to the Network's core competencies (Network for Social Work Management, 2019). Its Emerging Leadership Institute provides peer mentoring and coaching opportunities for early-to-mid-career professionals.

For such mentorship and training to happen, macro practice professors need to step up and step out (e.g., giving TED Talks, presenting at state and national conferences of practitioners, writing op-eds). We also need a national group of macro researchers to work with the Network for Social Work Management and the Association for Community Organizing and Social Action to more closely connect research to practice. And we may need to formalize the SSWR Special Interest Group on Organizations & Management Research so that it can support more regular professional development opportunities.

These developmental opportunities could be important because most schools do not regard TED Talks and op-eds as "scholarly works" even though they do represent thought leadership. Further, macro professors may overthink and "scholarize" public presentations because that is what they have been taught to do. Thus, they may overengineer their presentations through a scholarly, rather than a public, lens. It is not that the work is free from scholarship and evidence; it is based on those two legs. But professional communication should be accessible and inviting. To use one example, in scholarly work the conclusion usually comes at the end; in professional and policy communications it comes at the beginning. Hence, some of the organizations mentioned earlier might organize

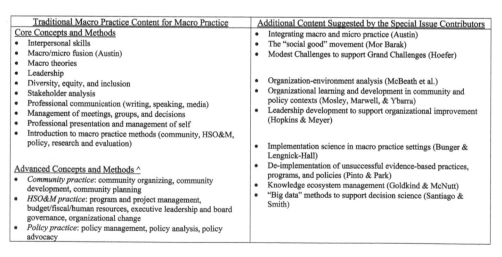

Traditional Macro Practice Content for Macro Practice	Additional Content Suggested by the Special Issue Contributors
Core Concepts and Methods • Interpersonal skills • Macro/micro fusion (Austin) • Macro theories • Leadership • Diversity, equity, and inclusion • Stakeholder analysis • Professional communication (writing, speaking, media) • Management of meetings, groups, and decisions • Professional presentation and management of self • Introduction to macro practice methods (community, HSO&M, policy, research and evaluation) **Advanced Concepts and Methods ^** • *Community practice*: community organizing, community development, community planning • *HSO&M practice*: program and project management, budget/fiscal/human resources, executive leadership and board governance, organizational change • *Policy practice*: policy management, policy analysis, policy advocacy	• Integrating macro and micro practice (Austin) • The "social good" movement (Mor Barak) • Modest Challenges to support Grand Challenges (Hoefer) • Organization-environment analysis (McBeath et al.) • Organizational learning and development in community and policy contexts (Mosley, Marwell, & Ybarra) • Leadership development to support organizational improvement (Hopkins & Meyer) • Implementation science in macro practice settings (Bunger & Lengnick-Hall) • De-implementation of unsuccessful evidence-based practices, programs, and policies (Pinto & Park) • Knowledge ecosystem management (Goldkind & McNutt) • "Big data" methods to support decision science (Santiago & Smith)

Figure 1. Traditional macro practice content and proposed content.

HSO&M = "human service organizations and management". ^ = Advanced research and evaluation content should be infused in all advanced macro practice content.

webinars to help macro professors develop the skills as well as comfort levels in carrying out their roles as public intellectuals.

What could the macro practice curriculum contain?

All 10 commentators dedicated attention to the question of future curricular emphases for HSO&M practice. They offered directions for the design and delivery of new macro practice courses, including leadership evaluation, the management of information ecosystems, data science, implementation science in relation to evidence-informed practice, organizational change through learning organizational approaches, and environmental justice, among others. Not only do these suggest important emerging foci, but they also reveal – singly and severally – how turgid and old school much of our curriculum has become.

Given their different foci and pathways of macroscopic interest, the macro practice areas displayed in Figure 1 might have some commonalities but also many differences of topic. The curricular map is meant to be illustrative and suggestive only, as many of the offerings in one pathway may be open to others. This curriculum would be fairly standard with some first year and/ or generalist practice content that would be largely required for all MSW students, but with some customization for schools that have specific macro majors rather than a general one.

Several curricular questions/issues will be asked by social work deans, directors, faculty, and students most notably. First is the sheer size of the MSW curriculum in a typical 60-credit hour program, especially when 25% of it is centered in field practica. Given concerns with student debt and time-to-completion as compared to other master's programs, it would be difficult to argue that MSW curricula should require more coursework and student credits.

A second issue concerns the conflation of interpersonal (group and team-based) and intrapersonal (i.e., clinical and direct practice) skill building. We would argue that interpersonal skills – including presentation of self and use of emotional intelligence, careful attention to cultural humility and evidence-informed practice, and the successful development and sustainment of groups in complex organizational and community settings – help micro and macro students alike. But they are not clinical skills as such. They are professional essentials for all fields of practice and professional roles.

A third is our general understanding that the rigor of social work courses at all levels could be, and should be, ramped up intellectually. Social work has often privileged feelings over facts, emotion over evidence, and interpersonal foci over intellectual ones. It is not that the second of each of these pairs of terms is absent; it is that they should not be subdominant. Indeed, "I feel" is altogether too common in social work macro practice, as opposed to "I think" or "In my judgment". The laxity of the former mode of professional discourse means that it is not possible to challenge someone's feelings in the same way that one can challenge one's conclusions based upon logical operations involving assumptions, conditions, premises, and expectations. For this reason, spirited macro practice discourse based upon ethical and evidentiary challenges may be somewhat muted.

As we strengthen the current offerings and add new macro content, we should also think about "de-traditionalizing" the workplace destinations of our graduates. Most of them go to traditional social service agencies. But macro content can also apply to many governmental departments at every level of government. Furthermore, there are corporate positions for macro practice graduates as well. Triple bottom line businesses (i.e., that emphasize profit, people, and the planet) would have spaces for them. Some corporations (e.g., Zappos, Tom's Shoes) have a social responsibility arm built directly into their business model. Departments of large corporations (e.g., human resources; diversity, equity, and inclusion) also are possibilities to be considered – not for everyone but for some.

How might an innovative school of social work "de-traditionalize" its macro practice concentration, by connecting course content and professional practice more intentionally? One might seek to reorganize the educational enterprise as follows: Each entry cohort of macro practice students would begin with four terms of coursework. Then students would be placed in a year-long paid formal internship with appropriate macro practice supervision and mentoring. The experience would culminate in a capstone followed by graduation and professional licensure. Such a proposal may seem radical from the perspective of social work educational accreditation. However, this proposal is similar to the structure of U.S. graduate medical education (with its two years of coursework followed by practice-based learning) (Accreditation Council for Graduate Medical Education, 2018).

Why is there less investment in research on HSO&M?

There is plenty of organizational scholarship and research. A back-of-the-envelope review of Google Scholar identifies 866,000 entries concerning organizational research and scholarship. There is ample, but less, intentional research on organizational research and scholarship for HSO&M. That said, the utilization of existing research and the production of research within the field may be lacking. For example, research by Google on the determinants of team excellence (called "Project Aristotle" in reflecting Aristotle's quote that the whole is greater than the sum of its parts) and managerial excellence (called "Project Oxygen") is not considered research by many scholars. Work by Gallup on the managerial determinants of strengths-based organizational cultures (Gallup, 2019) may be similarly disregarded.

Several intersecting reasons may provide a partial understanding.

Limited supply of prospective Ph.D. students

One can begin with the observation that there are only 77 Ph.D. programs in US schools of social work (CSWE, 2016). Ph.D. programs would naturally be a main source of HSO&M research done by social workers. However, many schools of social work have limited doctoral faculty and students.

The clinical preferential

Given the overwhelming dominance of clinical/direct practice at the master's level, we can assume that there would be a similar dominance in the Ph.D. area, except for those schools that have a significant proportion of macro practice faculty. For students to learn the craft of social work research, it is necessary to have faculty and doctoral students in sufficient quantity. As aforementioned, many schools are limited in macro professors and students at the advanced level.

Expectation differences between researchers and practitioners

For HSO&M researchers, subjects are organizations and those within them. Organizations do things; organizational researchers study how, when, why, where, and with what effects organizations do what they do. Managers regularly need to move quickly; researchers often choose to move more slowly and deliberately. Practitioners want answers, whereas researchers search for explanations. In addition, managers suggest that their agencies hold a "treasure trove" of data, while researchers suspect that they have a "messy field" of data. Fundamentally, organizational leaders and researchers may come from different structures and cultures. Each may become exasperated with the other.

Professional isolation

Few social work researchers can attend multiple conferences, so most attend the one that allows them to network with like-minded colleagues from different institutions. As a result, research conferences such as those held by business schools and industrial/organizational psychology departments (e.g., the Academy of Management) see relatively few social work attendees.

Collaborative impediments

This professional isolation is often mirrored on campus as well. Research and scholarship are most frequently a collaborative effort. However, there are serious barriers to collaboration among social work researchers and other researchers at most universities. Joint appointments in disciplines and in other professional schools with social work faculty generally exist only in the largest programs and in R1 universities. Logistical issues are a problem as well, with differing academic schedules. In many cases, schools of social work are located at some physical remove from other parts of the campus, creating geographical distance that may reinforce social distance between and among collaborators.

Differing perspectives concerning research evidence in social work and HSO&M

It may not be the absence of available research as much as the distribution, presence, and use of research that is more of an issue. Given the emotion, feelings, and interpersonal focus of social work, research may not rise to the top of one's mind, even though it is available. Research courses are among the least popular in most schools of social work – an attitude that may suffuse to the profession itself.

While there is a relatively recent call for evidence-based practices and interventions, important questions – such as how much evidence and what constitutes evidence, as noted in the commentary by Mosley, Marwell, and Ybarra – remain largely unanswered. Additionally, evidence-based initiatives are being replaced with a more flexible term of evidence-informed initiatives. And finally, much of the HSO&M literature remains at the useful-but-exploratory stage. Therefore, bench-to-bedside efforts to translate research and evaluation knowledge to organizational practice remain unavailable.

What can be done?

Here again, responsibility and accountability lie with past and present leadership of deans, directors, CSWE, and the professional practice community. Few real-world examples exist of academic-HSO&M practice partnerships, although some basic frameworks have been proposed (Austin, 2018; McBeath et al., 2019). In addition, macro practice faculty leaders should be added to the mix. For example, the SSWR Special Interest Group on Organizations and Management Research is an example of collective action on an inter-university basis. If it were given needed support, the Special Interest Group could be expanded to create additional opportunities for collaboration and professional development. Finally, opportunities exist within our journal to publish Learning from the Field cases. These cases provide opportunities for executives and scholars to feature examples of promising macro practices. Occasional sections of the journal could include brief interviews with prominent executives on novel practice topics.

Emerging problems and prospects in HSO&M research

Earlier in the essay, we briefly mentioned some knowledge gaps. Some additional absences stand out that deserve attention: problems of leadership and governance involving executive-board development and assessment. These issues concern the behavior of organizations and behavior in organizations. The first involves wrong-doing (or non-doing) at the organizational level, where the organization is a problematic actor (Greve, Palmer, & Pozner, 2010; Palmer, 2012). The second involves individuals in organizations acting badly. And the third is a combination of the first two concerns, in which the board and the C-level team collude in creating a culture of non-improvement.

This third concern involves social neutrality or "social bad", as opposed to "social good" (as Mor Barak encourages us to consider in her commentary).

Some of these concerns involve ethical lapses. Some lapses involve organizational leadership. Others of these concerns involve insufficient recruitment, education, training, and mentoring of boards of trustees. The human service sector does not have a robust talent management development system for the governance cadre. Few boards provide regular trainings for new board members and evaluations of their executive directors. Many violate their own bylaws, and retain trustees long after their "use by" date. Many are creatures of the CEO and exhibit only modest independence, if that. Rich 360-degree feedback and systematic evaluations of the CEO are often nonexistent.

The governance system is thus very loosely coupled from its formal duties and from the human service organization. All governors benefit from basic education, training, and evaluations of their board. The corporate sector has the periodical *Directors and Boards*, but there is no analogous publication for human service trustees.

Thus, research is desperately needed to fill the knowledge gap. From a macro practice research and education perspective, we need to embrace "the good, the bad, and the ugly".

Conclusion

We hope that this discussion of the special issue, illuminating as it does many areas of attention needed in HSO&M research and macro practice education and training, can serve as something of a wake-up call to the social work and human service organizational community that the sector is in grave danger. Concerns with the governance of agencies and the minimalistic attention to leadership and management training (both degree-based and post-degreed) suggest that the quality of our services is under threat, as is the field itself and the role of social work in it. Additional concerns with the diffuse state of macro social work researchers, and with the clear desire to enhance and reconfigure macro practice education, suggest that calls for more macro practice researchers and educators should be accompanied by evidence of return on investment in schools of social work. Strong, collective responses to these challenges are necessary from councils of deans and directors, collaborative professional development partnerships by leading and early career scholars supported by SSWR and CSWE, and associations of public and private human service organizations.

Disclosure statement

No potential conflict of interest was reported by the authors.

References

Accreditation Council for Graduate Medical Education (ACGME). (2018). *Engaging each other: Transformation through collaboration.* ACGME Annual Report 2017-2018. Chicago, IL: Author.

Austin, M. J. (2018). Mack center on nonprofit and public sector management in human service organizations. *Research on Social Work Practice, 28,* 386–391. doi:10.1177/1049731517710327

Council on Social Work Education. (2016). *Annual statistics on social work education in the United States.* Washington, DC: Author.

Flexner, A. (1915, May 12–19). *Is social work a profession?* National Conference of Charities and Corrections, Proceedings of the National Conference of Charities and Corrections at the Forty-second annual session held in Baltimore, Maryland, Chicago, Hildmann.

Gallup. (2019, September 11). *Manager development.* Retrieved from https://www.gallup.com/workplace/216209/develop-managers-leaders.aspx

Greve, H. R., Palmer, D., & Pozner, J. E. (2010). Organizations gone wild: The causes, processes, and consequences of organizational misconduct. *The Academy of Management Annals, 4,* 53–107. doi:10.1080/19416521003654186

McBeath, B., Mosley, J., Hopkins, K., Guerrero, E., Austin, M., & Tropman, J. (2019). Building knowledge to support human service organizational and management practice: An agenda to address the research-to-practice gap. *Social Work Research, 43,* 115–128. doi:10.1093/swr/svz003

Network for Social Work Management. (2019, September 11). *Competencies*. Retrieved from https://socialworkmana ger.org/competencies/

Nonprofit Academic Centers Council. (2019, September 11). *NACC membership*. Retrieved from http://www.nonpro fit-academic-centers-council.org/membership/

Palmer, D. (2012). *Normal organizational wrongdoing: A critical analysis of theories of misconduct in and by organizations*. New York, NY: Oxford University Press.

Specht, H., & Courtney, M. E. (1995). *Unfaithful angels: How social work has abandoned its mission*. New York, NY: Simon and Schuster.

Index

Note: **Bold** page numbers refer to tables; *italic* page numbers refer to figures and page numbers followed by "n" denote endnotes.

9 780367 495329